EAT LIKE A
WOMAN

(...and never diet again)

EAT LIKE A WOMAN

(...and never diet again)

A 3-Week, 3-Step Program to Finally Drop the Pounds and Feel Better Than Ever

Staness Jonekos
with Marjorie Jenkins, M.D.

*To the trailblazers who embraced the science of sex differences
and transformed the way we approach women's health.*

*And to my dad, who is somewhere between God and a rainbow.
You never told me how to live; you just lived showing me that anything
is possible. Thank you for always believing in me. I miss you every day.*

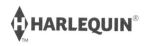

EAT LIKE A WOMAN

ISBN-13: 978-0-373-89269-3

The health advice presented in this book is intended only as an informative resource guide to help you make informed decisions; it is not meant to replace the advice of a physician or to serve as a guide to self-treatment. Always seek competent medical help for any health condition or if there is any question about the appropriateness of a procedure or health recommendation.

A full list of references used in the writing of this book can be found at www.eatlikeawoman.com.

Library of Congress Cataloging-in-Publication Data
Jonekos, Staness.
Eat like a woman: a 3-week, 3-step program to finally drop the pounds and feel better than ever / Staness Jonekos with Marjorie Jenkins, M.D.
pages cm
Includes index.
ISBN 978-0-373-89269-3 (pbk.)
1. Women--Nutrition. 2. Reducing diets--Recipes. 3. Exercise for women. I. Jenkins, Marjorie. II. Title.
RA564.85.J6152 2013
613.2'5--dc23
2013035214

www.Harlequin.com

Printed in U.S.A.

CONTENTS

Chapter 8

Eat This or That? Food Controversies

Chapter 9

Eating Strategies for a Healthy Weight

*When women demand equal care, we declare our
equal capacity to contribute fully to society. When we learn
about and value our bodies, we become truly powerful.*

*A woman who says with conviction,
"My health is worth fighting for," is saying, "I am worth fighting for."*

—Bernadine Healy, M.D.

INTRODUCTION

ARE YOU EATING LIKE A MAN?

It all began 8 years ago when I gained 25 pounds in a short period of time as I slammed into menopause unprepared. My health and sanity were being chipped away from age-related conditions such as high blood pressure, a slowing metabolism and out-of-whack hormones. My self-esteem and youth were swept off in an avalanche of misery and confusion.

Doctors and experts had no real solution for me. Some gave me medications, others encouraged me to take a vacation, and a few even suggested unproven remedies that did not work and only worsened my condition. I tried every diet known to *man* with no success. I was desperate to lose weight and start to feel normal again.

I decided to conduct extensive personal research using myself as a human guinea pig, tweaking the FDA's food pyramid recommendations for carbohydrates, protein and fat. The result? I hit the weight-loss jackpot. I lost 25 pounds in 12 weeks! Once I adjusted my proportions of protein to carbohydrates to fats and incorporated some other important lifestyle habits, I was able to achieve a healthy weight. I felt better, I looked better and my health improved.

Everyone asked for my secret, so I wrote *The Menopause Makeover*, and teamed up with leading menopause expert Dr. Wendy Klein.

Something amazing happened when the book hit the stores—word spread that the book's recommendations were not only helping women who were experiencing the various stages of menopause, but that the food program I had designed was also helping women of *all* ages find their healthy weight. I got e-mails from women worldwide thanking me for a plan designed especially for women. The stories were remarkable and inspirational. Women struggling to lose baby fat after childbirth successfully lost weight. Perimenopausal women got control over their symptoms and achieved their ideal weight again. Postmenopausal women who had never reached a healthy weight were able to slip into their college-sized clothes for the first time in decades.

What made this new program work for women of all ages? The understanding that women and men are different! The program in *The Menopause Makeover* embraces a woman's unique metabolism, recognizes the biological and emotional differences between men and women, and honors the nutritional needs of women—which I discovered applies to women at each life stage.

Readers asked me why *The Menopause Makeover* program was limited to just one life transition, so I developed an easy-to-use program designed for women of any age to get healthy, lose weight and lead a more balanced life.

The Journey to *Eat Like a Woman*

My journey began searching for a scientific reason that supported my food formula. Properly trained by Dr. Wendy Klein, co-author of *The Menopause Makeover*, I knew where to find the latest science. She opened the golden gates to the Society of Women's Health Research, a leader in sex-based research, and it all started making sense. My food program worked because women are very different than men—from our brains to our guts to our hormones.

Sounds logical, right? Here is the shocking part. Incredibly, many of our medical treatments and dietary solutions have been derived from the biology and physiology of a man! Yes, it's true. For decades, research was conducted using only men, even when studying the risks and benefits of menopausal hormone therapy! Therefore, what we know about women's nutrition has largely been based on the typical 70-kilogram man, long used in medical science as a reference standard. Only recently has research focused on a woman's biology and physiology, with the results slowly trickling into the mainstream.

However, many current best-selling diet books continue to present programs for men and women that are based on the research results that used men only and ignore the critical fact that men and women are different, making the assumption that men and women will benefit from the same plan. Bewildering, isn't it? It's no surprise that many women complain about their men losing more weight on the same diet. So if you've struggled on other diets and nutrition programs and wondered why, the answer may be a simple one: you're not a man!

I was surprised and a bit furious that the medical field was thousands of years behind the times when it came to women's health, and even more upset when I learned women still have not received equal attention as men. Equality in this sense is not "men and women should be medically treated the same"—rather, it is taking into account that women and men are different and that differences matter. Growing up as part of the first generation of women to have the right to design our lives—career, motherhood and closer to equal pay (at $0.78 to the dollar for women, this area still needs work)—I was naive to think the medical world granted equal health rights. It is shameful that women's health has been marginalized medically and politically, but tragic that inequality in health still exists between women and men.

Fortunately, some incredible people sounded the alarm, and changes started happening over the past two decades that required researchers to include women as subjects and state whether or not this had been done. Supporting the health of all women is imperative to paving a future of wellness, regardless of ethnicity, socioeconomic status or geography. If our sisterhood is to be strong, it will take all of us walking the same path with the same goal—women's health for all.

This book is a road map through the maze of weight gain frustration for all women.

This book is possible because visionaries have made a commitment to include women in research and to incorporate the results of that research into medical schools and mainstream practice. Both women and men should receive equal attention in the medical community. We must recognize that when it comes to men and women, differences matter, whether it is in heart disease, osteoporosis, Alzheimer's disease or breast cancer.

The sex and gender differences acknowledged in this book are the latest as of publication. True, we don't have all of the answers. After all, men have been studied for thousands of years, while women have been included only for a few years. Some of what we discuss in this book can be applied today, while other concepts may need continued research. As we collect more data over time, individualized treatments and personalized medicine for both women and men will be possible.

Dr. Klein introduced me to Marjorie Jenkins, M.D., who is the chief scientific officer of the Laura W. Bush Institute for Women's Health at Texas University Health Sciences. Dr. Jenkins, a former chemical engineer, was drawn to women's health as she became aware of the discrepancies in the way women's health issues were addressed and treated, and the gap of knowledge about women's health in the medical literature. She is committed to evidence-based medicine that incorporates the differences between men and women. We were both on the same mission—an awareness campaign about the different health needs of women and men! And so our journey together began.

Dr. Jenkins's enthusiasm about gender-specific women's health and her vast expertise has helped me build a strong scientific foundation for *Eat Like a Woman*. When we had conversations about the content of this book, I always learned new things—and then I would often become angry when I realized that so few of us have access to this information. Now you have this incredible new science at your fingertips. It is only the beginning of a long journey, but the past 20 years have yielded some discoveries that will astonish you and have you asking, "How could the scientific world think we were just like men? Did they really think the ability to have children, breastfeed and have a menstrual cycle were the only differences between men and women?"

Just recently at a doctor's appointment, I was asked about my latest projects. When I told him I was writing a book that applies the latest science on sex and gender difference to a woman's lifestyle program, he looked at me and said, "Other than pregnancy, what differences from men are there that can be applied to a lifestyle program?" And at that moment I knew I was on the right path with the right partner in the creation of the Eat Like a Woman program and the writing of this book.

The *Eat Like a Woman* Approach

Ladies, you will be among the first to read about the latest science that explores our amazing differences. *Eat Like a Woman* takes this incredible information and applies it in an easy-to-use 3-step, 3-week program.

Part One of this book shares the latest science on why you should eat like a woman, celebrating the many differences between men and women, from our hormones, brain, digestive system and fat cells. Part Two reveals the components of the *Eat Like a Woman* 3-week program. Part Three gives you the tools to eat like a woman for life, including wonderful *Eat Like a Woman*–approved recipes from our favorite celebrities and chefs. What are they eating to maintain health? What are their guilty food pleasures and advice?

Step 1 of *Eat Like a Woman* is the foundation of the program; you will learn how to eat like a woman for each life stage. Whether you are a vegetarian, vegan or omnivore, you will find solutions that fit with your preferred lifestyle choice.

Step 2 embraces that emotional health is very different for a woman than a man. This step will open the door to your unique essence of being, so you can nurture healthy emotions and create a life in balance.

Step 3 supports your fountain of youth, but you will have to SWEAT for it! **S**mart **W**omen **E**xercise **A**ll the **T**ime! With modifications for each life stage, Step 3 will give you tips to fuel fitness for life.

A list of all references used during my research for this book, as well as health calculators, recipes, products and services to start eating like a woman, can be found at www.eatlikeawoman.com.

No matter what life stage you may be in today, your lifestyle and genetics can determine your risk of disease, and being a woman affects susceptibility to disease and responses to dietary treatments. Therefore, sprinkled throughout the book are tips on how you can prevent, manage and treat disease with lifestyle choices. In general, women have different nutrient requirements and respond differently to drugs, so disease prevention and management is different. Food, in fact, is the number one preventative weapon against disease, so reducing risk and managing disease with proper food choices through the *Eat Like a Woman* program can add years to a woman's life.

It is not too late to start embracing your body, your womanhood, and your right to celebrate that you are different! This book will give you tools so you can go out into the world and demand individualized care, personally, medically and politically.

It's Time to Eat Like a Woman

I have written *Eat Like a Woman* because we *must* change how we think about food and embrace our bodies as women. I have written *Eat Like a Woman* for women who, just like me, want to have a fulfilling life supported by good health, good food and good times. I have written *Eat Like a Woman* because it is time we all celebrate womanhood and our unique relationship with food. When it comes to health and nutrition, sex differences matter, and that fundamental fact is at the heart of *Eat Like a Woman*.

Eat Like a Woman is for women with busy lives, and since the program was inspired by my own personal struggles, I'm a perfect example of the life-changing results that are possible. I have practiced and benefited personally from what is written in this book. Because the program has its origins based on the eating plan in *The Menopause Makeover*, it is endorsed with incredible testimonials from women of all ages at different life stages. Once you make the simple lifestyle changes outlined in *Eat Like a Woman,* your quality of life can improve, and the many transitions you will go through as a woman may be less dramatic.

The late Bernadine Healy, M.D., former head of the National Institutes of Health (NIH), once said, "Nutrition is undoubtedly the single biggest factor influencing the health and well-being of women at any stage of life." Therefore, this book is packed with food lists, weight-planning tools, meal planners, activity charts and sample food plans, all supported by the latest sex-based research. *Eat Like a Woman*'s 3-step plan is a vital blueprint for life that can change the way women eat, and holds the key to being happy in your own skin, adding years to your life.

Eat Like a Woman boldly goes where no diet book has gone before—to a new frontier where women eat like women and refuse to choose the "gender-neutral" diet plan. I was liberated knowing that new, exciting sex- and gender-based science is in the pipeline. It is my hope that this book's scientifically sound message will allow you to look at your body and weight in a new and exciting way.

While *Eat Like a Woman* guides you to healthy eating and exercising based on the evidence that women and men are different, it also celebrates a woman's emotional and spiritual relationship with food. This important connection can fuel good or bad eating habits that affect our health and self-esteem. In these pages, we will tackle the stresses associated with appearance and body image, showing you how to build confidence and a sense of self-worth.

Science + Women's Health = Eat Like a Woman

This program will help you:

+ Maintain a healthy weight effortlessly.
+ Focus on your future, not your weight.
+ Be as healthy at age 50 as you were at age 25.
+ Slide through each life stage with ease.
+ Reduce your risk of disease.
+ Slow the aging process.
+ Understand how stress is related to health and disease.
+ Understand your neurotransmitters so you know what messages they are sending about your health.
+ Learn the basic idea behind the design of the woman's body.
+ Discover how your hormones work and how they control your body in each life stage.
+ Learn how hormone imbalances can cause many health problems and how they can be corrected without medication.

This program embraces that we are all different and that women are not simply smaller versions of men. Sex matters.

The message is simple: *eat like a woman,* and you will obtain your healthy weight and improve your health for life. Can you eat like a man? Sure! But if you want to honor your body, don't eat like a man—*eat like a woman!*

1

Why You Need to Eat Like a Woman

Chapter 1

The *Eat Like a Woman* Formula for a Healthy Life— and the Science Behind It

- Did you know it takes women's stomachs an hour longer than men's to empty after eating?
- Did you know that women's bodies are much more efficient at grabbing carbohydrates from foods before digesting protein and fat?
- Did you know that women taste food differently?
- Did you know that nutrients are absorbed more slowly as they pass through the gastrointestinal tract in women compared to men?
- Did you know that the government's national dietary standards—the recommended daily allowances (RDA) that you see on nutritional labels—were originally based on the studies of young healthy male World War II military recruits?
- Did you know that prior to the 1990s the most popular research subject was the "70-kilogram [154-pound] white man"?

As discussed in the introduction, nutritionally and medically, women have historically been treated like smaller versions of men. In fact, until recently, most research studies did not even consider that there might be sex- or gender-based differences in health and disease, and research efforts and approaches to health and wellness were based on the male model. Yet the science of the past two decades has revealed more about the differences between men and women. As a result, the scope of women's health has expanded beyond a narrow focus on those things that affect only women—pregnancy, menstruation, menopause—and now addresses how women in particular are affected by diseases that impact men and women, such as heart disease, cancer and osteoporosis, rather than excluding women from these studies.

Fortunately, we have the opportunity to now make health decisions based on the female model. In *Eat Like a Woman,* I have taken this new research and applied it to a woman's life, creating a program designed for women that embraces each life stage, so you can maintain good health at your healthy weight for life. However, this level of attention to the unique health needs of women and the inclusion of women in clinical research is a relatively recent advancement in science.

Women's Health Is a Woman's Right

The field of nutrition, women's health and the women's movement have had critical intersections over the past 150 years. One focus of the early suffrage movement was women's health. At the time, women could not gain access to information about contraception and were banned from most medical studies. It was thought that only by gaining the right to vote could women have some say about their own bodies.

While women battled for their rights, nutrition as a modern science was born in the early 1900s with the discovery that food contained specific vital nutrients, such as proteins, carbohydrates, fatty acids, vitamins and minerals.

At this time, the National Institutes of Health (NIH, then a small laboratory), was focusing on a deadly disease called pellagra that deteriorated the skin, gut and brain. They discovered that this disease was not a mental condition nor communicable but actually a dietary deficiency, and pellagra was wiped out with nutritional adjustments. The association between nutrition and the prevention or curing of disease propelled the scientific field of nutrition.

Ellen Swallow Richards, the first woman to study for a Ph.D. at the Massachusetts Institute of Technology in 1876, founded the nutrition and home economics movement in the United States. Female scientists committed to women's health and nutrition found a safe harbor in home economic departments. Two leaders of the home economics field, Lulu Graves and Lenna Cooper, founded the American Dietetic Association (ADA), now called the Academy of Nutrition and Dietetics, in response to the nutritional needs of soldiers in World War I.

The terms *sex* and *gender* are often used interchangeably in literature. In accordance with the Institute of Medicine, I use the term *sex* when referring to the biology of a female or male as determined by the individual's genes and hormones. I use *gender* when referring to a person's self-representation as female or male, and how a person is viewed in society and his or her environment.

Despite the initial positive movement of nutritional science, this new field was inadequately funded by congressional and university budget committees that were composed mostly of men. Both female and male research scientists were wary about devoting a lifetime to the field of nutrition. Nutrition in the form of home economics persisted but was marginalized or ignored by mainstream scientific researchers. Condescendingly, home economics began to be known as the "Mrs. major."

Though advances in understanding the role of nutrition in health continued, women's health suffered a major setback in 1977 when the Food and Drug Administration (FDA) barred women of childbearing age from participating in most early-phase clinical research. Supporters of this action claimed the FDA's intention was to protect the fetus and possibly avoid liability. Critics claimed it was to prevent women from freely choosing to participate in research.

In the early 1980s, the Congressional Caucus for Women's Issues, a group of female U.S. congressional representatives, announced that it appeared that the medical research community had been ignoring women's unique health needs. Throughout most of the twentieth century, research into diseases that affect both men and women often included only male participants. As a result, the understanding of women's health and nutrition suffered. In 1985, the United States Public Health Service Task Force concluded that the exclusion of women from clinical research was detrimental to women's health.

In 1986, the NIH adopted guidelines urging for the inclusion of women in NIH-sponsored clinical research. Despite this urging, important research was still being done using only men. According to Susan Calvert Finn, Ph.D., R.D., F.A.D.A., former president of the American Dietetic Association, in the 1980s there were studies on the effect of estrogen as protection against heart disease, and the research was done using *men*. Research during that time also explored the effect of obesity on the development of breast or endometrial cancer, and again that research was conducted using *men*. Studies of the relationship between vitamins and cancer were conducted using only *men*.

Fortunately, the 1990s brought together government, health-care institutions, academia and advocacy organizations to promote women's health. In 1990, the Society for Women's Health Research (SWHR) was founded, and they asked the General Accounting Office (GAO) to examine whether the NIH was following its 1986 guidelines. The GAO report revealed that the NIH guidelines were not being followed, citing the Physician's Health Study or "aspirin" study, which was designed to examine the effect of taking aspirin on cardiovascular disease. This massive study included no women.

That same year, the NIH strengthened its guidelines and established the Office of Research on Women's Health (ORWH) to focus on ensuring women's participation in clinical trials and to promote the career advancement of women in science. However, decades of clinical studies that focused mainly on the "70-kilogram man" had left a void of female-based data in all areas of research, from nutrition studies to treatments for diseases.

As a direct result of the efforts of women's health advocates, the Women's Health Initiative was launched in 1991. This 15-year, $625 million NIH study was the largest clinical research study of women and their health ever undertaken in the United States or elsewhere. This study involved 161,808 generally healthy postmenopausal women.

The NIH Revitalization Act of 1993 mandated that no clinical trials on human subjects would be government funded unless they included women and minorities. Around this same time, the FDA withdrew its earlier guidelines barring the participation of women of childbearing age from most early-phase research.

Women's health was once again on the radar. President Clinton mentioned women's health research as a national priority in his 1994 State of the Union address soon after First Lady Hillary Clinton, who headed up the Task Force on National Health Care Reform, remarked upon "the appalling degree to which women were routinely excluded from major clinical trials of most illnesses." Major medical centers established special programs in women's health that included more than reproductive health as their focus.

Over 20 years after the Congressional Caucus for Women's Issues blew the whistle on the medical research community for ignoring women's unique health needs and over 10 years after the GAO concluded that the NIH was not effectively monitoring research data to determine how sex and gender differences affect drug safety and effectiveness, many well-respected organizations saw the need to focus on women's health needs. In 2004, the Academy of Nutrition and Dietetics (formerly the ADA) and the Dietitians of Canada published a position paper that strongly supported research, health-promotion activities, health services and advocacy efforts that would enable women to adopt desirable nutrition practices for optimal health. Their position statement acknowledged that women's health-related issues were multifaceted, and that nutrition had been shown to greatly influence the risk of chronic disease, as well as assist in maintaining a woman's optimal health.

Research on women's health has seen unprecedented growth over the past two decades, and the more we include women in research studies, the more we find that there are significant differences between men and women. Women are not smaller versions of men, and differences matter. That is what *Eat Like a Woman* is about.

Today, women's health is recognized as a national priority. Continued success depends on political commitment; sufficient funds; interested scientific communities; advocacy by professionals; and the involvement of women, men and communities working for equality and recognition of sex differences.

Recently I had the privilege to meet Vivian Pinn, M.D., the former director of the Office of Research on Women's Health (ORWH) and the former codirector of the Women's Health Initiative. A true pioneer, she was the only woman and only African-American in her medical school class and has dedicated her life to women's health. I asked Dr. Pinn what action women can take to ensure the progress of women's health, and she answered:

> *The current political environment, which sometimes has personal biases based on religion, based on culture, based on naivete, is affecting the ability of women to get the types of health care that they need. Having women informed, women asking questions of their health-care providers, that will really be a major influence in changing how medicine is practiced.*

As you read *Eat Like a Woman* and apply the information to your own life, discuss this new sex-based science with your doctor. Those questions will be our bridge between research and reality.

Just this past decade there has been an increase in studies and campaigns promoting women's health awareness, ensuring safer and more effective use of medicines, and evaluating strategies to achieve healthful behaviors—improved diet, nutritional supplementation, increased physical activity and early disease detection—for women of all races and ethnic groups at all life stages. We have all benefited from the efforts of our foresisters who fought for our rights and advances in women's health, but we must continue to have our voices heard. Women's unequal treatment affects our well-being and lives in many ways. The women's movement—fighting for the same political, economic and social rights as men—has been and will continue to be an important part of women's health.

Does Sex Matter?

Thanks to the efforts of the ORWH, the NIH, and the SWHR, regulations and guidelines have been changed to include women in research studies. In April 2001, the U.S. Institute of Medicine (IOM) announced publication of a landmark report, *Exploring the Biological Contributions to Human Health: Does Sex Matter?* This report validated the scientific study of sex difference as a means to improving health. Fortunately, since this report was issued, interest in sex-based science has increased. Thus, in the 21st century, it has finally been formally acknowledged that, yes, sex matters.

The unique combination of genetic, hormonal, and physiological traits of women affects your susceptibility to disease and how your body responds to dietary treatments. What you eat, what you do for fitness, and how you manage stress can help you reduce your risk and help manage disease, as well as maintain a healthy weight.

The differences in a woman's brain, hormones, digestive tract, body composition, and life stages make us unique, and it starts in the womb. Sex differences begin at the time of fertilization, depending on whether an egg is fertilized with a sperm carrying an X or a Y chromosome. These differences continue to manifest throughout the life span.

Thousands of genes behave differently in females and males. This explains why the same disease often strikes females and males differently, and why the different sexes may respond differently to the same drug or dietary intervention. However, despite the measureable differences between males and females in more than half of the genes' expression patterns, both sexes have genes that are turned on and off by regulatory genes. Regulatory genes are controlled mainly by nutrients. This means that just because your parents had weight issues does not mean you will have weight issues. Similarly, if heart disease runs in your family, proper nutrition and a healthy lifestyle can indeed reduce or eliminate your risk. There is no question that genetics are a factor, but your health destiny can be influenced by nutrition.

Before we move forward with the *Eat Like a Woman* program, let's review the latest discoveries about our sex differences. Make a note of what applies to your life. In Step 1 of this book, foods that reduce risk or manage certain conditions will be presented so you can customize your program.

According to the SWHR, there are some areas in which women's bodies and health differ significantly from men's.

- ♦ ADDICTION: Women are more likely than men to experience severe withdrawal symptoms when trying to quit an addictive substance, and they generally find it more difficult than men to quit.

- ♦ ALCOHOL: Women produce less of the stomach enzyme that breaks down ethanol, a type of alcohol found in alcoholic beverages. After consuming the same amount of alcohol, women have a higher blood alcohol content than men, even after adjusting for size.

- ♦ AUTOIMMUNE DISEASES: More women than men suffer from autoimmune diseases such as multiple sclerosis, rheumatoid arthritis and lupus. Lupus and fibromyalgia are nine times more common in women than men. Rheumatoid arthritis is two to three times more common in women.

- ♦ BRAIN: Females have a larger deep limbic system, the area of the brain that is associated with being able to express feeling and bonding. The areas in the frontal temporal lobes of the brain that are related to language are larger in women, explaining women's superiority in language skills over men.

- ♦ CANCER: Cancers of the lungs, kidneys, bladder and pancreas are more common in men; thyroid and breast cancer are more common in women.

- ♦ CORTISOL LEVELS: Women react more quickly than men, so we have higher levels of cortisol, the stress hormone. Higher levels of cortisol not only trigger appetite, but they can also encourage deposition of fat in the abdomen.

- ♦ DEPRESSION: Women are two to three times more likely than men to suffer from depression. A woman's brain synthesizes neurotransmitters—chemicals important to mood and function—differently than a man's. This difference contributes to a woman's risk of being depressed because her brain makes less serotonin, a neurotransmitter.

- **DIGESTION:** A woman's stomach responds differently than a man's when digesting a meal. We take almost an hour longer than men to empty our stomachs. Women are much more efficient at grabbing every bit of carbohydrate from the foods we eat before we digest protein, increasing our ability to store fat. Nutrients and drugs are absorbed more slowly in women than in men as they pass through the gastrointestinal tract, bloating and belching are more common in women, and female kidneys are slower to act than male kidneys.

- **DRUG REACTIONS:** Many common drugs, like antihistamines and antibiotics, cause different reactions and side effects in women than in men.

- **ENERGY METABOLISM:** Women, on average, have lower energy expenditure than men, mainly as a result of differences in the body composition.

- **FAT CELLS:** Females are born with billions more fat cells than males. The fat cells in an adult woman's body are five times larger than a man's, which means there is more room for storage.

- **HEART DISEASE:** More women than men die from heart disease. Men experience heart attacks, on average, ten years earlier than women and have a better one-year postattack survival rate than women. Symptoms of heart attack show distinct gender differences: most men experience acute, crushing chest pain, whereas most women experience shortness of breath and fatigue, as well as chest pain. Women have fewer strokes but are more likely to die from them than men; women are generally older than men when they have a stroke. Today, researchers say when men have heart disease it affects the larger blood vessels, but in women, the small blood vessels become diseased.

- **HORMONES:** A woman's sex hormones are obviously very different than a man's (more in Chapter 2).

- **IMMUNE FUNCTION:** Women are usually less likely to develop infections (except with AIDS) and more likely to develop autoimmune diseases. Hormones produced by the ovaries for women and testicles for men markedly affect immune and inflammatory cell responses.

- **IRRITABLE BOWEL SYNDROME (IBS):** Women are two to three times more likely to develop IBS than men.

- **LEPTIN LEVELS:** Leptin is a hormone produced by the fat cells that controls appetite, energy and metabolic rate. Women tend to have more fat cells than men, and they generally have higher leptin levels. New studies show that leptin might reduce anxiety and improve depression in women.

- **MIGRAINE HEADACHES:** Postpubescent women are more than twice as likely as men to suffer from migraine headaches.

- **OBESITY:** Extreme obesity is more common in women than men. Puberty, pregnancy and menopause are significant factors in the development of obesity in women.

- OSTEOPOROSIS: Women comprise 80 percent of the population suffering from osteoporosis.
- PAIN: Some pain medications, such as kappa opiates, are far more effective in relieving pain in women than in men.
- SMOKING: Smoking has a more negative effect on cardiovascular health in women than in men.

As you can see, from our genes to our hormones to how we digest food, there are substantial sex differences.

At least some of the health issues that women are particularly vulnerable to can be favorably influenced by nutrition. For example, following a low-fat, vegetarian diet can reduce menstrual pain and premenstrual stress (PMS) symptoms. Conversely, there is a negative relationship between alcohol consumption and breast cancer risk. As few as three drinks a week are associated with an increased risk of breast cancer.

In 2001, SWHR held a briefing on Capitol Hill to discuss the IOM's report entitled *Exploring the Biological Contribution to Human Health: Does Sex Matter?* Mary-Lou Pardue, Ph.D., chair of the IOM committee that published the report, said: "Sex does matter. It matters in ways that we did not expect. Undoubtedly, it also matters in ways we have not begun to imagine." Therefore, the time has come for an up-to-date program that recognizes these fundamental differences between the sexes, so women can take control of their health and happiness with a lifestyle that supports a woman's body for a lifetime. Today, the results of the Women's Health Initiative discussed previously, the largest clinical study ever undertaken by the NIH in the 1990s, are still being interpreted and being applied to clinical practice.

As we gain a deeper understanding of sex-based science, the current results of the latest research suggest that nutrition is probably the single biggest factor in the health and well-being of a woman at any stage of her life. In a 1997 commentary that appeared in the *Journal of the American Dietetic Association,* Susan Calvert Finn, Ph.D., R.D., F.A.D.A., former president of the ADA, said, "Nutrition is at the forefront of women's health and holds the key to the prevention and treatment of the most devastating diseases that affect women and their families."

The *Eat Like a Woman* program is supported by the latest sex-based science embracing your unique biology and physiology. This 3-step program can be applied at every life stage from puberty to menopause with appropriate nutritional and caloric variations. Women have four distinct life stages that are accompanied by physiological, psychological and biochemical changes, so an alteration in the daily intake of nutrients is required.

What we eat can change our health profile and quality of life. The *Eat Like a Woman* 3-step program will give you tools to incorporate healthy habits into your life. It is never too late to start eating like a woman.

The Mind-Body-Spirit Connection

Humankind has acknowledged through the ages that the way we feel can influence our bodies, as the mind-body-spirit connection has been observed since ancient times. Today, there are many researchers trying to see just how our thoughts, attitudes, beliefs, emotions and health affect each other for both sexes. Scientists have now developed a new branch of medicine to explore the link between emotions and the immune system called psychoneuroimmunology (PNI), confirming that our emotional and spiritual health are directly related to physical health.

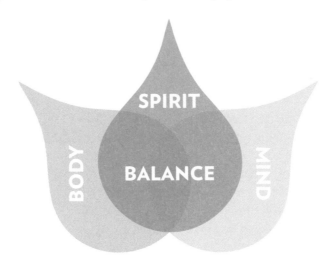

FORMULA FOR A HEALTHY LIFE

Balanced Mind + Body + Spirit = Good Health

Just as our bodies and minds are very different than a man's, our formula to maintain health through each life stage needs to be different, too. Although both sexes need to give attention to their mind, body and spirit in order to obtain good health and find balance in life, a woman's physiological and psychological differences are very real, from genetics to hormones to body composition. Finding this balance requires a different strategy for women than for men.

There have been times in my life where I experienced great emotional stress, and my physical health inevitably paid the price. After caring for my father while he was dying of brain cancer, not only did I look 10 years older, but my overall health was a disaster. My blood pressure was sky-high, I was depressed, my allergies flared up, I could not sleep, my stomach was constantly upset, I felt tension in my chest, I got headaches, and I lived in a constant state of irritability and anxiousness. Feeling hopeless, I started drinking a couple of glasses of wine or vodka on the rocks at night to find peace. When that did not work, I added Benadryl so I could sleep at night. I could only hope the passage of time would return my sanity and health. For me, the evidence that our mind, body, and spirit are connected had never been stronger.

Most of us have experienced how our emotions influence our health, but are the body and mind distinct from each other, or do they function together as part of an interconnected system? Searching for more than personal validation, I went on a quest for a scientific answer. After digging through numerous scientific journals, I discovered a study published in the *Journal of Immunology* conducted by neuroscientist Candace B. Pert, Ph.D., former chief of brain biochemistry at the National Institutes of Health. Pert's results confirmed that the mind and body are indeed connected.

According to Pert, the neural, hormonal, gastrointestinal and immune systems are equipped with neuropeptide receptors and the capability to produce neuropeptides. (Neuropeptides are molecules that allow neurons to communicate with each other.) This network connects the major systems of the body so that cellular signals between mind and matter are translated into physical reality. For example, stress and depression can physically suppress the activity of lymphocytes, the white blood cells that are the body's first line of defense against cancer and invading organisms. In addition, neuropeptides cause chemical changes in the body that can improve or weaken the immune system.

How does this mind-body evidence apply differently to a woman's journey versus a man's? During the past two decades, new science has acknowledged that a woman's brain, hormones, neurotransmitters, and digestive and immune systems are very different from a man's. Our emotions and the resulting chemical reactions in the body will affect us differently, too.

Let's use stress as an example to demonstrate how the mind, body and spirit are all interconnected. We'll start with the brain's response to stress. Many things can fuel stress, and stress has many negative effects. Women have a deeper limbic system than men. The limbic system is a complex set of brain structures that supports emotions, behavior, motivation, long-term memory and sense of smell. The deep limbic system of females is larger than that of males, and is associated with women being able to express their feelings and be more in sync with their feelings than men. This also helps with bonding to others, an evolutionary maternal benefit. A larger, deep limbic system combined with our ever-changing sex hormones can trigger emotions, and, in turn, emotions can ignite an avalanche of anxiety, pumping our bodies with cortisol, the stress hormone.

Neuroscientists say the changes in the brain during stress response last longer in women because of this larger limbic system. This physical occurrence, coupled with the fact women produce less serotonin, the happy neurotransmitter, can make women two to three times more prone to depression than men (more in Chapter 3). In addition, high cortisol levels coupled with low serotonin levels can lead many of us to search for carbs that help flood the brain with tryptophan, an amino acid that converts into serotonin, so we feel better. Low serotonin levels are also associated with a decreased immune system function.

Stress can also affect your sleep. In turn, sleep deprivation can increase cortisol levels, which can cause fat accumulation in the lower abdominal area and affect your ability to control your mood and make good decisions.

Have you ever felt that you weren't just "clicking on all cylinders"? Coauthor Dr. Jenkins tells me that women sometimes think they are getting Alzheimer's or some other memory disease when really they are just stressed out! Recent studies conducted by Larry Cahill, Ph.D., a professor of neurobiology and behavior at the University of California at Irvine, revealed that stress hormones interact with sex hormones. When women had high levels of estrogen before and during their periods, acute stress blurred their recollection abilities.

Living on an emotional roller coaster, no thanks to ever-changing hormones and a deeper limbic system, can hijack your physical and psychological health (it certainly did for me). These physical sex differences combined with a woman's busy day-to-day stressors, such as juggling family and career, can make having good health a struggle.

As women, managing our emotional health is critical to obtaining physical health, and both are fueled by our belief system. When something bad happens, how you interpret the situation comes from your belief system. Do you see stressors as meaningful events that are connected to your individual life purpose, finding lessons to improve your quality of life? Or do you approach challenging situations with resistance and anger, increasing stress levels? Our modern world is full of daily stressors for both men and women, but women are often the ones responsible for both managing finances and family. With a strong belief system, a woman's spirit can fuel a healthy connection between the body and mind.

Why Most Diet Plans Fail

A recent survey estimated that 108 million Americans are dieting. It is no surprise the dieting industry is a $65 billion industry and continues to grow. Forbes analyzed the cost of about a dozen popular diets and found the average diet costs 50 percent more than what an average American spends on food!

However, many diet plans today do not embrace a woman's unique mind-body connection and how a woman's composition differs from a man's. Have you ever gotten frustrated when you did not see immediate weight-loss results after starting a diet? That frustration can create stress, and those stress hormones can actually lead you to further gain weight rather than lose it—leading to depression and compromising your immune system.

It is no surprise that women begin the unhealthy process of yo-yo dieting, which can compromise their heart health and immune system and promote more weight gain on each rebound. Leading obesity expert, Kelly D. Brownell, Ph.D., director of the Rudd Center for Food Policy and Obesity at Yale University, who coined the term "yo-yo dieting" in the 1980s, says, "Weight cycling can actually change your physiology. So the more diets you've been on, the harder it gets to lose weight. A hunger hormone called ghrelin increases, and a fullness hormone called leptin decreases, so you feel hungrier and less satiated."

According to the National Eating Disorder Association, a leading non-profit organization in the United States, in the last 10 years:

- About 70 percent of adult females have been on a diet. One in three women are on a diet at any given time.
- Between five and ten million women and girls have struggled with eating disorders and borderline conditions. Only one million boys and men struggled with eating disorders and borderline conditions.
- The "typical" dieter has started up to four diets a year.
- More than 80 percent of people who have lost weight have regained all of it or more after two years.

In the past few decades, the majority of adult women in the United States have been on a diet because the female population overall is getting heavier. Women are consuming a lot more calories than they did just 30 years ago. By the year 2000, women ate the equivalent of one cheeseburger every day—that's 335 more calories—compared to what they ate in 1971, according to a study by the Centers for Disease Control and Prevention. Today, 90 percent of online dieters are women. The most common starting weight class is now 175 to 199 pounds, surpassing the 150- to 174-pound class for the first time since 2005. The average waist size was 28 inches 60 years ago. Today it is 34 inches! What has changed since then?

- Both women and men have become more sedentary because technology has replaced physical activity. We sit at a computer all day, sit on the couch with a remote control watching TV, play video games and spend time commuting in a car. Studies show the average American spends an average of 4.5 hours a day sitting in front of a television, computer or video game.
- Fast food is too convenient, too available.
- Fast food or junk food is often cheaper than healthful organic foods.

- A busy lifestyle contributes to increased stress, and that can lead to emotional eating.
- The convenience of processed food has overshadowed our desire to prepare meals with fresh foods.
- The media has planted an unhealthy expectation that women must be skinny to be attractive. Unable to obtain "skinny status," many become depressed, and the emotional eating roller coaster begins.
- Many food businesses are producing unhealthy food products injected with high-fructose corn syrup.
- Large portions are served in restaurants. The average entree could feed a family of three!
- There are fast-food restaurants inside some schools. Fast-food chains are showing up in airports, malls and, yes, even hospital cafeterias.
- Technology has isolated individuals, so food can provide comfort for loneliness. Who hasn't binged on a pint of ice cream while watching TV after a bad day?
- When we don't have a healthy self-esteem and serotonin levels are low, women tend to reach for high-glycemic carbs (cookies, French fries) for relief.
- With the deep and prolonged recession, people have turned to lower-priced fast and comfort food.

Perhaps a combination of culprits may be fueling the obesity epidemic that is forcing our population to search for diet solutions. If you picked up this book because you are struggling to obtain a healthy weight, what are the contributing factors? Are you too busy to think about nutrition? Do you buy fast food because it is cheaper? Is your self-esteem low? Are you feeling hopeless?

What Can We Do Differently?

I believe the key to solving the global obesity epidemic starts with women.

- We must make responsible health decisions for each life stage. The decisions that seemed right in our teens may not be right in midlife.
- We must demand that health-care providers view our needs through a gender-neutral lens.
- We must make changes that contribute to lifelong health.
- We must properly feed our bodies, nourish healthy emotions and celebrate our spirituality.

The *Eat Like a Woman* health formula embraces the sex differences with a unique 3-step plan designed just for women that builds a foundation for finding balance between the mind, body and spirit at each life stage so we can achieve and maintain a healthy weight for life.

Using this formula, the *Eat Like a Woman* program lays out a system that you can automatically access for help with incorporating a lifestyle that supports balance as a woman.

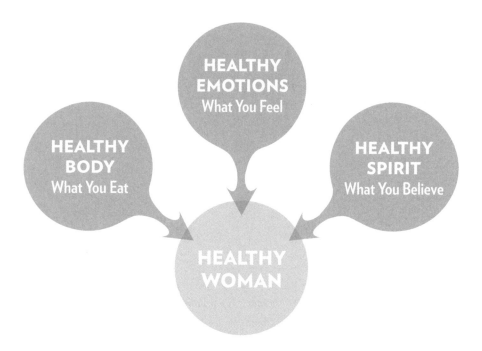

From our brains to hormones and neurotransmitters, women differ greatly from men. You must create balance between the mind, body and spirit to achieve health. Making time to nurture healthy emotions, being informed, fueling a healthy body with the correct food choices and daily activity, and nourishing your spirit are all necessary to honor your overall health and happiness.

You cannot focus on one portion of the formula and expect lasting success. You can eat perfectly and exercise daily, but if you are depressed, maintaining this commitment will be challenging. If you don't give time to your belief system, feel alone and respond to challenges with anger, you may not have the motivation to eat well and exercise. All areas must be balanced to support healthy lifestyle choices.

If you are wondering how I pulled out of my declining health situation after my dad passed away, I can tell you that this 3-step prescription saved my physical, emotional and spiritual health.

Worry, stress, anger, guilt and fear are negative emotions that can influence your immune system and create inflammation, contributing to disease. Hypertension, allergies, infections and autoimmune diseases can all be fueled by unhealthy emotions. Low self-esteem can lead to obesity. Obesity can lead to type 2 diabetes and heart disease risk. All areas of your life must be in balance to be well. What you feel emotionally becomes your physical reality.

Balance is the key to the *Eat Like a Woman* plan. If you have healthy eating and exercising habits but are riddled with toxic emotions, you increase your risk of disease. If you live a perfectly peaceful and spiritual life but eat junk food, you compromise your health. We must weave all aspects of our life together to create overall health. The human spirit must be strong to battle the mind's war games so the body stays healthy.

Chapter 2
Hormones:
Your Brain-Body Connection

Let's start by taking a simple quiz.

YES	NO	SYMPTOM
		Are you depressed?
		Do you struggle with your weight?
		Do you crave sweets?
		Are you hungry all the time?
		Do you have mood swings?
		Do you have abnormal facial hair?
		Do you get migraines?
		Do you suffer from persistent breast tenderness?
		Do you have frequent gas and bloating?
		Do you bruise easily?
		Do you cry for no reason?

continued on page 24

YES	NO	SYMPTOM
		Do you have water retention?
		Do you have brittle nails?
		Do you have difficulty falling asleep?
		Do you have irregular periods?
		Do you have a decreased libido?
		Do you have excessive thirst?
		Do you suffer from hot flashes?
		Do you get fatigued easily?
		Do your joints and muscles ache?
		Do you feel dizzy and weak?

If you answered yes to any of these questions, your hormones may be out of balance.

Hormonal Madness

How many times have we blamed hormones for how we feel? I have suffered from hormonal imbalances my entire life, as did my mother, her sister and their mother.

My loving parents had to live through my erratic, moody teenage years. I had heavy periods coupled with awful PMS, and I suffered from terrible allergies. My doctor at the time told me that my hormonal imbalances were caused by school pressure or by moving every other year as an Air Force "brat." I was promised I would grow out of it. Those were the days when so many experts told women, "It's all in your head."

These imbalances affected my daily life. The school nurse would send me home because I used to faint when my periods were heavy. I had to use a tampon of the highest absorbency level and two super-sized pads, so wearing the tight, sexy hip-hugger jeans that were in style those days was impossible. It was an embarrassing and confusing time. My mother was very understanding and gave me the tools to survive because she, too, suffered from heavy periods. This nightmare ended

30 years later with a terrible menopausal experience that included a 25-pound weight gain and hourly hot flashes.

During these frustrating and formative years of my own growing up, the whole notion of women's health was coming into focus. Today, we can benefit from the intervening years of research into women's unique hormonal health.

We now know that both sexes produce the same hormones but in differing amounts and differing patterns. More than 50 different hormones have been identified in the human body, and more are still being discovered.

Hormones and the glands that secrete them influence and regulate practically every cell, tissue, organ and function of our bodies, including growth, development, metabolism, digestion, sleep, sexual and reproductive function, and how we absorb fat. Hormones contribute to our weight and how we handle stress. Hormones can influence what the brain is interested in doing and your daily behavior, such as feeling flirty, wanting to cuddle or have sex, nurturing your loved ones, and wanting to feel attractive. In essence, hormones are the vehicles of the brain-body interaction—an important foundation of the mind, body and spirit connection.

Once a hormone is secreted, it travels from the endocrine gland through the bloodstream to target cells designed to receive its message. Think of it as a lock and key: the cell is the lock, and the hormone is the key that unlocks a specific pathway that is needed for us to feel healthy and energetic.

Hormones influence our emotions, but our emotions can also influence our hormones. Add in physical symptoms and erratic moods, and—voilá!—you are in the middle of a hormonal imbalance. Dr. Jenkins calls this the "Her-mood-al cycle."

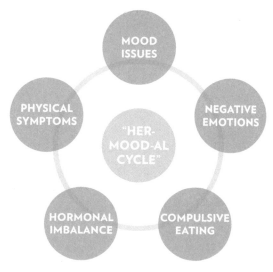

Source: M. Jenkins, M.D. Used with permission.

When we talk about hormones, you may think of estrogen and progesterone, but there are many other hormones in our body.

Estrogen regulates energy expenditure, appetite and body weight. Having insufficient estrogen receptors in specific parts of the brain can lead to obesity. Estrogen produced by your endocrine system weighs no more than a miniscule microchip, yet your daily estrogen level can have a huge effect on how you feel.

What we eat, our level of activity and our overall outlook on life can greatly influence the health of the glands and organs that produce our hormones. Many blame thyroid issues for weight gain, moodiness on our sex hormones and fatigue on our adrenals, but a minor change with one gland can affect the entire endocrine system. Supporting the health of your endocrine system is important. If there is an imbalance of hormones secreted from one gland, it can affect the levels of hormones secreted from the other glands.

When we feel bad and are stressed and those stress hormones pump out, we turn to chronic junk food consumption, which, in turn, can lead to hormonal chaos. When you over-consume high-glycemic carbohydrates such as desserts or potato chips, the body's insulin levels rise and you store fat. Manage insulin levels with proper food intake, and you are on your way to a healthy weight.

The Happy Home of Hormones

The *Eat Like a Woman* program is designed to promote hormonal health. I will make references to different hormones during the *Eat Like a Woman* 3-step plan in Part Two of this book, so let's take a journey through our endocrine system, your home of hormones.

♀♂

The hormone leptin is found in our fat cells. Leptin tells the body when we are hungry and when we are full, and it also regulates energy intake and expenditure. When levels are high, it signals the brain that we are full and can stop eating. Women have different leptin levels than men, and since women have more fat cells than men, it is no surprise that our leptin levels are different. When you lose weight quickly, your leptin levels fall, you get hungrier and metabolism drops. That is why quick weight-loss diets are not good for you, and many women begin yo-yo dieting.

THE ENDOCRINE SYSTEM

The Hypothalamus: Hormone Headquarters
Connects the nervous system to the endocrine system via the pituitary gland. Regulates hunger, thirst, fatigue and body temperature.

The Pituitary Gland: Queen of Glands
Produces hormones that control functions of other endocrine glands, including the release of thyroid hormones. Triggers ovulation, kick-starts lactation, induces contractions during labor, stimulates water retention, maintains muscle mass and fat distribution, influences growth, and regulates your period and metabolism.

The Thyroid: Metabolism Mama
Regulates metabolism, controlling how fast the body breaks down food. Plays a role in the bone growth and development of the brain and nervous system in children.

The Pancreas: Sugar Beware
Produces insulin, which controls blood sugar levels, and enzymes and hormones, which help break down food.

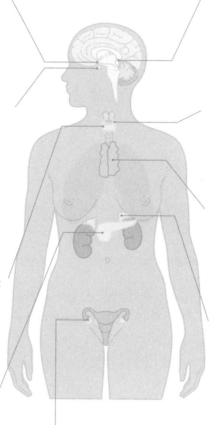

The Pineal Gland: Sleeping Beauty
Regulates the sleep-wake cycle and body temperature. Affects estrogen, progesterone and testosterone levels signaling menstruation and affects the start of menopause.

The Parathyroids: Bone Buddies
Regulate calcium levels in the blood and bone metabolism. Calcium maintains the electrical energy in the nerves, providing muscles with energy.

The Thymus: Immunity Warrior
Promotes production and maturation of white blood cells that protect the body from certain threats, including viruses and infections.

The Adrenal Glands: Stress Manager
Produce hormones that help the body respond to stress and danger. Also regulate the body's metabolism, the balance of salt and water in the body, and blood pressure.

The Ovaries: A Lifelong Journey of Change
Produce hormones involved in reproduction. Regulate menstruation and gestation.

Endocrine glands and endocrine-related organs are like mini-factories, each producing and storing hormones and releasing them as needed. There are many factors that affect endocrine function:

- Aging
- Illness
- Chronic or acute conditions
- Infection
- Autoimmune destruction
- Traumatic injuries
- Surgery

- Cancerous and noncancerous tumors
- Birth or genetic defects
- Stress
- External factors
- Genetics
- Environmental factors/toxins
- Poor lifestyle habits

> All steroid hormones, including cortisol, estrogen, progesterone and testosterone, are made from cholesterol. Your body manufactures some cholesterol and your diet provides the rest.

Managing your emotions, nutrition, and stress, and avoiding external toxins, can contribute to a healthy endocrine system.

Now let's take a look at various components of the endocrine system and how they affect your body.

The Hypothalamus: Hormone Headquarters

The hypothalamus is located in the brain and is the primary link between the endocrine and nervous systems. It regulates hunger, thirst, sleep, body temperature, appetite, sexual behavior and reproduction, neurotransmitters, and blood pressure. It also secretes hormones that will increase or decrease the release of other hormones in the pituitary gland.

The hypothalamus also keeps track of estrogen (estradiol) in the body. When levels get low, the hypothalamus sends an order to the pituitary gland telling it the body needs more estrogen.

The hypothalamus is an organ with significant sex differences. The area of the hypothalamus involved with mating behavior is 2.2 times larger in men than in women and contains twice the number of cells.

Anorexia, bulimia, malnutrition, head trauma, radiation, surgery and too much iron can cause hypothalamic dysfunction. Because of the interrelatedness of the glands in the endocrine system mentioned previously, hypothalamic disease can have a negative impact on the pituitary glands, which can ultimately affect the thyroid glands. Avoiding malnourishment and excessive iron through a well-balanced diet can contribute to hypothalamic health.

The Pituitary Gland: Queen of the Glands

The pituitary gland is referred to as the master gland. I call it the queen of all the other glands, although it is no bigger than a pea. It is located at the base of the brain, just beneath the hypothalamus, and controls biochemical processes important to our well-being.

As the master gland of the body, it produces and secretes many hormones that travel throughout the body, directing certain processes that stimulate other glands to produce different types of hormones.

The pituitary gland makes these hormones:

◆ ADRENOCORTICOTROPIC HORMONE (ACTH): ACTH stimulates the production of cortisol by the adrenal glands. Cortisol, the "stress hormone," is vital to our survival. It helps to maintain blood pressure and blood glucose levels.

◆ ANTIDIURETIC HORMONE (ADH): ADH, also called vasopressin, regulates water balance.

◆ FOLLICLE-STIMULATING HORMONE (FSH): FSH stimulates the ovaries to enable ovulation. LH and FSH work together to cause normal function of the ovaries.

◆ HUMAN GROWTH HORMONE (HGH): HGH stimulates growth in childhood and is important for maintaining a healthy body composition and well-being in adults. In adults, it is important for maintaining muscle mass, bone mass and fat distribution in the body, and it strengthens our immune system.

HGH peaks during the teen years and slowly declines as we get older. Many people think that supplementing their diet with HGH in the form of pills, powders and injections will help them lose weight, as it helps build muscle mass and reduce body fat, but HGH is not a dieter's solution, nor is it safe! HGH supplementation is not an effective treatment in obese people, and the American Association of Clinical Endocrinologists has warned that the use of HGH for obese patients is not recommended.

◆ LUTEINIZING HORMONE (LH): LH helps regulate the menstrual cycle and causes ovulation.

◆ PROLACTIN: This hormone stimulates milk production in the breasts after childbirth. It also affects sex hormone levels in the ovaries.

- **THYROID-STIMULATING HORMONE (TSH):** TSH stimulates the thyroid gland, which regulates the body's metabolism, energy, growth and nervous system activity. This is the "fuel" hormone.

- **OXYTOCIN:** This hormone is known as the "hormone of love" because it is involved with lovemaking, fertility, contractions during labor and birth, and the release of milk in breastfeeding. If oxytocin production is not working optimally and an individual has an oxytocin deficiency, then she may be prone to postpartum depression, generalized depression and anxiety, social isolation, phobias, panic attacks, sleep difficulties, and other common stress-related ailments.

The pituitary gland functions as the thermostat that controls all other glands responsible for hormone secretion. This gland is a critical part of our ability to respond to the environment, most often without our knowledge.

Pituitary disorders can have a major effect on a woman's menstrual cycle. When the pituitary causes too much prolactin to be produced, a woman can experience irregular menstrual cycles or a lack of periods altogether. Too much prolactin can also cause a woman's breasts to produce a discharge that resembles milk.

Women create 60 percent more prolactin than men. Prolactin levels increase with stress and can create the response of emotional tears, as opposed to tears that flush an irritant out of your eye. Humans are the only species that have emotional tears. A lot of emotional crying may be a signal that your stress levels are at an unhealthy level.

The Pineal Gland: Sleeping Beauty

The pineal gland is a pinecone-shaped gland of the endocrine system that is located in the middle of the brain and is only the size of a grain of rice. The pineal gland produces several important hormones, including melatonin.

Melatonin influences sexual development and regulates the sleep-wake cycle, body temperature and cardiovascular function, and it is a derivative of the amino acid tryptophan. (Tryptophan is needed for the body to produce serotonin, and melatonin is made from serotonin.) Melatonin levels can affect your estrogen, progesterone and testosterone levels, which, in turn, signal menstruation and affect the start of menopause. Melatonin also affects insulin production.

The pineal gland's production of melatonin is dramatically increased during nighttime hours and falls off during the day because melatonin is also produced in the retina (light-sensitive tissue

♀♂

When women are under stress, the hormone oxytocin is released. This hormone causes us to gravitate toward "tending or befriending" — women feel the urge to tend the children or family or go see friends. This action of tending or befriending causes the body to release more oxytocin. Estrogen also enhances oxytocin and increases this oxytocin stress response, explaining a sex difference in the stress response.

Although men do produce oxytocin, the male hormone testosterone dampens the effect. This may explain why, when women are stressed, we call our friends or gather family around, but when men are stressed, they are more inclined to work things out on their own.

that lines the inner surface of the eye) by photoreceptor cells. The more darkness your eyes receive, the more melatonin is produced.

Our sleep cycle begins with the production of melatonin from the pineal gland. In the middle of the night, the hormone prolactin is secreted in large amounts. These two hormones promote an immune reaction that restores a healthy balance. This process also targets viruses, pathogenic bacteria, man-made chemicals and foreign proteins in the body.

For the necessary amount of melatonin and prolactin production to occur, you need eight hours of sleep. With inadequate sleep, these hormones are unable to effectively enhance immunity. There are also many melatonin-related disorders, such as stress, depression, sleep disorders, immunological disorders, cardiovascular disease and cancer.

The pineal gland may only be the size of a grain of rice, but the queen of the glands holds great power over our health, weight and quality of life. Melatonin production peaks around age 5, and by the age of 60, we will lose up to 80 percent of those original levels, so many of us won't sleep as well at that age. Do you recall how your grandparents would get up at the "crack of dawn"?

Melatonin is also produced in the gastrointestinal tract. The amount of melatonin in the digestive system is 400 times greater than in the pineal gland.

The Thyroid: Metabolism Mama

The thyroid, located in the front part of the lower neck below the larynx, is shaped like a bow tie or butterfly and produces the thyroid hormones thyroxine (T4) and triiodothyronine (T3). It plays an important role in the body's metabolism and has an effect on energy, growth and development, and nervous system activity.

Thyroxine is called T4 because it contains four iodine atoms and enters targeted tissues directly to assist with metabolic functions. T3 is actually T4 that is converted into a more useful form in the liver and other tissues, like the brain. T3 loses one of its iodine atoms during this process. Both T4 and T3 have similar functions stimulating and maintaining metabolic processes and are controlled mainly by the thyroid-stimulating hormone (TSH) secreted by the anterior pituitary gland.

Research shows there is a direct interaction of estrogen with the expression of thyroid-sensitive genes. Estrogen and other female hormones affect the regulation of the thyroid axis—comprised of the hypothalamus, pituitary gland and thyroid gland—which is responsible for metabolism. When hormones that affect metabolism are not functioning properly, a woman may either lose or gain weight.

The thyroid gland needs iodine to properly function and pump out thyroid hormones. Too little iodine and the thyroid can't make enough hormones, but too much iodine stops the thyroid gland from working.

*Hypo*thyroidism—too little of the hormones or a low-functioning thyroid gland—is the thyroid disorder most women are concerned about since it can cause them to gain weight. It can also make a person depressed and unresponsive. Too much thyroid hormone production, *hyper*thyroidism, can increase metabolism and cause weight loss, but it can also speed up the effects of aging and make you feel agitated or jumpy.

Women are 5 to 8 times more likely to develop thyroid disease than men because women have unique risks for thyroid disease. One of these is pregnancy, and a woman has a 10 percent chance of developing thyroid disease after pregnancy. Thyroid disease in adolescent girls has the ability to either delay their first menstrual period or bring it early. In adult women, the disease has the potential to adversely affect the menstrual cycle and fertility.

The table below outlines the differences in *hyper* and *hypo*thyroidism.

Hyperthyroidism	Hypothyroidism
Heat intolerance	Cold intolerance
Nervousness, irritability, heart palpitations	Memory loss
Light periods	Heavy periods
Insomnia	Fatigue, forgetfulness, difficulty concentrating
Increased appetite	Decreased appetite
Weight loss	Weight gain
Increased sweating	Decreased sweating
Brittle, thin hair	Hair loss, dry skin
Diarrhea	Constipation

Estrogen and progesterone can both stimulate thyroid inflammation since oral estrogen can affect thyroid hormone levels by increasing thyroxin-binding globulin. Women taking oral estrogen therapy or estrogen and progestins, including oral contraceptives, need to have their TSH level monitored and their dose of replacement thyroid hormone (levothyroxine) adjusted if needed. You should have your TSH level checked if you start having symptoms of hypothyroidism listed above.

The Parathyroids: Bone Buddies

Attached to the thyroid are four tiny glands that function as a unit, called the parathyroids. They release the parathyroid hormone (PTH), which regulates the level of calcium in the blood with the help of calcitonin, which is produced in the thyroid. Both the thyroid and parathyroid glands also play a role in the regulation of the body's blood calcium balance. Calcium maintains the electrical energy in the nerves and provides the muscles with energy, as well as maintains bone health.

If your calcium intake, calcium absorption efficiency or vitamin D levels go down, you don't absorb calcium as well. As a result, the PTH glands increase secretion to draw calcium from the bones and offset what would otherwise be a drop in blood calcium. When the parathyroid gland is stimulated to over-function, the condition is known as hyperparathyroidism and leads to hypercalcemia. For women, the prevalence of hypercalcemia increases thirty-fold after menopause.

The Thymus: Immunity Warrior

The thymus gland forms part of the immune system. It is situated in the upper part of the chest, behind the breastbone, and is made up of two lobes that join in front of the trachea. The thymus is an important part of children's immune systems. It enlarges from about the 12th week of gestation until puberty, when it begins to shrink. Thymosin is the hormone produced by the thymus. The main gland function is to produce and process lymphocytes, also known as T cells, which go to the lymph nodes (immune system cells) and protect the body from certain threats, including viruses and infections.

Most diseases of the thymus affect the immune system. Exercise daily to ensure that blood circulates throughout the body and the thymus. The increased blood flow will ensure that thymus waste products are removed promptly and do not cause damage to the thymus.

The Adrenal Glands: Stress Manager

Adrenal glands secrete hormones that help regulate chemical balance and metabolism and supplement other glands. The body has two triangular adrenal glands that perform very separate functions—the adrenal cortex and the adrenal medulla—one on top of each kidney.

The **adrenal cortex** is the outer portion of the adrenal gland, and its functions are necessary for life. The adrenal cortex secretes hormones directly into the bloodstream that have an effect on the body's metabolism, on chemicals in the blood and on certain body characteristics.

It was only recently that laboratory testing took into account that women's "normal" thyroid levels were not the same as men's. In fact, most of what was thought to be "normal" had been discovered from testing only adult Caucasian men. For years, many women thought they had low thyroid only to hear from their doctor that their levels were normal. The range of normal has been narrowed, but we still need more data to discover the optimal range of normal thyroid levels for women. For now, if you feel you have low thyroid symptoms you should discuss it with your doctor.

Among the hormones produced by the adrenal cortex are the corticosteroid hormones hydrocortisone (cortisol) and corticosterone. Hydrocortisone helps control the body's use of fats, proteins and carbohydrates. It is designed to be a short-term coping mechanism to deal with extreme stress. When cortisol levels are too high, the immune system is suppressed, and insulin, blood pressure and blood sugar levels increase, which may lead to brain damage. Corticosterone, combined with hydrocortisone, suppresses inflammatory reactions in the body and also affects the immune system.

Hormonal imbalance of the adrenals causes excess cortisol, creating chronic stress, and chronic stress leads to even more cortisol. Chronic stress is stress that lasts for more than three months. Juggling a busy life, work, family, finances, career, losing a loved one, caretaking or divorce can upset your hormone balance.

Aldosterone is also produced by the adrenal cortex. It controls sodium levels secreted into the urine and maintains blood volume and blood pressure.

Another product of the cortex is androgens, often called the "male hormones," and they affect the body's metabolism. The principal androgens are testosterone and androstenedione. Both women and men produce androgens, but in differing amounts. Men produce higher levels. In women, they are converted into the female hormones, estrogens. The ovaries and adrenal glands produce about 40 to 50 percent of the body's testosterone.

In adult women, androgens play a key role in the prevention of bone loss, as well as sexual desire and satisfaction. They also regulate body function before, during and after menopause. Excess amounts of androgens can cause excess hair growth, acne and thinning hair. High androgen levels can lead to insulin resistance and diabetes, high cholesterol, high blood pressure and heart disease. Low androgen levels can cause fatigue, decreased libido and susceptibility to bone disease. By the time a woman reaches menopause, her androgen levels have declined 50 percent or more, accelerating bone loss.

Another hormone, dehydroepiandrosterone (DHEA), is made from cholesterol by the adrenal glands and is the most abundant hormone found in the bloodstream. It is considered to be the mother hormone because it is used to produce other hormones such as estrogen, progesterone, testosterone and cortisol. Balanced levels of DHEA send messages to each of our 100 trillion cells to repair, rebuild, restore and revitalize. It also improves our memory, mood, immune system and longevity.

> DHEA supplements have been advertised to slow the effects of aging on muscles and the immune system. Researchers are working to find more definite evidence in order to determine if there is support for these claims. In the meantime, if you are thinking about taking DHEA supplements, be aware that the effects are not fully known and might turn out to cause more harm than good. Notify your primary care provider if you are thinking of taking DHEA supplements.

When the adrenal glands are chronically stressed, your production of DHEA can be greatly reduced. DHEA is a good stress barometer, because when stress levels go up, DHEA levels go down. Both DHEA and androstenedione can be converted to testosterone.

There are tests that can measure DHEA levels, and if they are markedly low in a fatigued woman, some health-care practitioners will provide short-term DHEA supplements. The bottom line is do not self-treat. As Dr. Jenkins says, "This hormone stuff is tricky, and you might cause more harm to your endocrine system."

The primary task of the **adrenal medulla** is stress management, but it is not necessary for life. The hormones secreted by the adrenal medulla include epinephrine and norepinephrine. Most people know epinephrine by its other name—adrenaline. This hormone rapidly responds to stress by increasing your heart rate and rushing blood to the muscles and brain. Also known as noradrenaline, norepinephrine is both a hormone and neurotransmitter, and it works with epinephrine in responding to stress. However, it can cause vasoconstriction (the narrowing of blood vessels), which results in high blood pressure.

The adrenal glands work hand-in-hand with the hypothalamus and pituitary gland. The interactions among these organs, called the HPA (hypothalamic-pituitary-adrenal) axis, are a major part of the nervous and endocrine systems that control reactions to stress and together they also regulate digestion, the immune system and emotions.

You may have heard of adrenal fatigue or read about it in magazines or online, but according to the Endocrine Society, adrenal fatigue is not considered to be a real medical condition, and there is no test that can detect this condition. Supplements and vitamins made to "treat" adrenal fatigue may not be safe. Taking these supplements when you don't need them can cause your adrenal glands to stop working and may put your life in danger.

The Ovaries: A Lifelong Journey of Change

Biological sex refers to the chromosomal complement that makes each of us uniquely a woman or a man. Two X chromosomes make us female, so let's find out how powerful our sex hormones are and how they influence each life stage.

Our sex hormones are primarily made in the ovaries, which are located on both sides of the uterus. The ovaries contain the egg cells necessary for reproduction, and they also produce

For a man, estrogen is testosterone's little sister. Men also produce estrogen but in much smaller amounts. Estrogen is produced in a man's adrenal glands and is controlled by the hippocampus section of the brain. Estrogen is critical for a man's brain function. Hmmmm, and we wonder why the sexes communicate differently.

estrogen and progesterone. Estrogen is required to form the ovum (egg) and prepares the uterus for implanting a fertilized egg.

Estrogen includes a group of chemically similar hormones. Estrone (E1) is made mainly in fatty tissue and the liver during menopause. Estradiol (E2) is produced in the ovaries, as well as in the adrenal glands and fat tissue during premenopause when levels start to decline. Estradiol is abundant during the reproductive years. Estriol (E3) is produced by the placenta during pregnancy and is the weakest of the estrogens.

In addition to being produced by the ovaries, estrogen is also produced by the body's fat tissue (more on this in Chapter 5). In women, estrogen circulates in the bloodstream and binds to estrogen receptors on cells in targeted tissues, affecting the breasts and uterus, as well as the brain, bone, liver, heart and other tissues.

Progesterone prepares the breasts for lactation during pregnancy and works with estrogen to regulate the menstrual cycle. In addition to being processed in the ovaries, progesterone is also produced in the adrenal glands and in the placenta during pregnancy.

Let's see the important roles estrogen and progesterone play in a woman's body.

ESTROGEN	PROGESTERONE
Decreases appetite and food intake	Stimulates appetite in the presence of estrogen
Decreases body weight and promotes distribution of fat in the butt and thighs	Increases body weight in the presence of estrogen
Helps preserve bone density	Is essential for fertility and ensuring a healthy pregnancy
In the brain, regulates temperature, memory and learning; increases cerebral blood flow; regulates sexual development and reproduction; has antioxidant and anti-inflammatory effects	Regulates monthly menstrual cycles if you are not pregnant
Stimulates breast development at puberty and prepares the glands for future milk production	Increases core temperature during ovulation

continued on page 38

ESTROGEN	PROGESTERONE
Helps regulate the liver's production of cholesterol—increases production of HDL (healthy) cholesterol and decreases LDL (bad) cholesterol	Protects and regulates brain activity
In the kidneys, affects salt balance and keeps blood pressure low	Helps reduce risk of osteoporosis by building bone mass
Stimulates the maturation of the ovaries, regulating menstrual cycles and reproduction	Reduces gallbladder activity
Increases body fat	Uses fat for energy
Increases collagen production that thickens the skin	Regulates blood sugar levels
Stimulates the maturation of the uterus and helps prepare the uterus to nourish a developing fetus	Aids in normalizing blood clotting
Helps maintain a lubricated and thick vaginal lining	Regulates the effects of estrogen on the uterine lining to safeguard it
Has an effect on dopamine, our reward and energy neurotransmitter	Contributes to initiating sleep
	Serves as a natural diuretic and antidepressant
	Has an effect on serotonin, our happy neurotransmitter
	Can help reboot libido
	Regulates thyroid hormone

Women also make testosterone in small amounts from the ovaries and adrenal glands. Most men produce 6 to 8 milligrams of the hormone testosterone (an androgen) per day, compared to most women who produce 0.5 milligrams daily.

A woman's testosterone level is highest around age 20 and slowly declines until it is half as high in her 40s. Testosterone boosts strength and increases lean body mass for women and men but there are sex differences. Testosterone actually increases appetite and food intake for women, and it promotes binge eating and can increase abdominal fat. However, it also increases muscle mass, metabolic rate and red blood cells, and it promotes strong bones. Testosterone initiates protein synthesis and promotes the release of growth hormones released from the pituitary gland during deep sleep.

In women, testosterone may be linked to sex drive. But for women, interest in sex is much more complicated than just testosterone levels. Feeling unattractive, not being happy, being fatigued, or suffering from vaginal dryness can all contribute to a woman's libido.

A recent review on sex hormones, appetite and eating behavior in women says sex hormones play an essential role in the regulation of appetite, eating behavior and energy metabolism. Food intake and reproductive functions are closely related, so it is no surprise that our daily food intake varies at different hormonal phases during the menstrual cycle. Women tend to eat less during the early part of the menstrual cycle before ovulation takes place, when estradiol levels are high. It is also the time when women are more sexually receptive and active. When progesterone levels are high, food intake is increased.

Women eat more during pregnancy to ensure normal growth of the fetus, and it is suspected that higher levels of progesterone that occur during pregnancy are responsible. The influence of both estrogen and progesterone is that fat is deposited in the butt and thighs so there is an energy reserve during breastfeeding. During menopause, declining estrogen levels are associated with more abdominal fat. This may explain why hormone therapy actually lowers weight gain and body fat for many women.

Keeping Your Endocrine System Healthy

The endocrine system is like a beautiful orchestra with many players that need to play on key to be enjoyed. With just one out-of-tune player, the entire performance can go out of tune. Let's look at the things we can control, such as lifestyle choices, and things we cannot control, such as age, so we understand the importance of good daily habits to increase the odds of hormone balance.

Sex hormone levels can be affected by the following:

* Hypogonadism
* Hypopituitarism
* Pregnancy failure (estriol)

+ Perimenopause and menopause (estradiol)

+ Polycystic ovarian syndrome (PCOS)

+ Anorexia nervosa (eating disorder)

+ Extreme exercise or training

+ Estrogen levels that rise during a healthy pregnancy

+ Increased estrogen levels that may be seen with tumors of the ovaries, testes or adrenal glands

+ Low levels of estrogen immediately after childbirth and also during breastfeeding

+ Steroid medications, ampicillin, estrogen-containing drugs, phenothiazines and tetracycline, which can increase estrogen levels

+ Ulcer medications (cimetidine), clomiphene (a selective estrogen-receptor moderator used as a fertility drug), some antibiotics (erythromycin and clarithromycin), antifungal medications, medications for thyroid disease and certain antidepressants such as Prozac, which can affect estrogen levels; these medications and many other medications that are used by women can interfere with the effects of estrogen on tissues and the levels of estrogen achieved in the bloodstream, so it is important to discuss your prescription medications and over-the-counter supplements with your health provider

+ Marijuana and cocaine, which can affect estrogen levels

+ Fat cells have the ability to produce an enzyme known as aromatase; this plays a role in converting testosterone into estrogen, thus changing the hormonal balance

+ Certain tumors of the adrenal and pituitary glands, and the liver and lungs, as well as liver disease, high blood pressure, kidney disease and thyroid disease, which may elevate estrogen levels

+ Caffeine and alcohol, which can both alter estrogen levels

+ Certain pesticides, chemicals and herbicides, which have the potential to cause estrogen-like effects in the body

+ Hormone-enhanced food products, which raise estrogen levels

With all the factors that can affect our sex hormones, it is no surprise that maintaining a healthy weight can be challenging for women. Puberty, pregnancy and menopause are significant factors in the development of obesity in women, suggesting that fluctuations in reproductive hormone concentrations uniquely predispose women to excess weight gain.

Use this summary of the female hormones as a quick reference if you have a concern about your personal health and to prepare for your next doctor's appointment.

SUMMARY OF FEMALE HORMONES

GLAND	HORMONE	ACTION
Hypothalamus	Regulatory hormones of anterior pituitary hormones	Acts on anterior pituitary to stimulate or inhibit hormone production; plays a major role in the regulation of appetite and food intake
Pituitary Gland	Oxytocin	Stimulates the mammary glands to eject milk during lactation and the uterus to contract during childbirth
	Antidiuretic hormone (ADH)	Stimulates water resorption by kidneys; acts on the arteries, promoting their contraction; acts on the kidneys, preventing water excretion
	Human growth hormone (HGH)	Stimulates body growth, fat breakdown and formation of antibodies; reduces body fat; strengthens bones and immune systems
	Prolactin	Promotes lactation
	Follicle-stimulating hormone (FSH)	Stimulates follicle maturation and production of estrogen
	Luteinizing hormone (LH)	Helps regulate the menstrual cycle and causes ovulation

continued on page 42

GLAND	HORMONE	ACTION
Pituitary Gland (continued)	Thyroid-stimulating hormone (TSH)	Stimulates release of T3 and T4
	Adrenocorticotropic hormone (ACTH)	Promotes release of glucocorticoids
Pineal Gland	Melatonin	Regulates sleep
Thyroid Gland	T3 (Triiodothyronine) & T4 (Thyroxine)	Stimulates metabolic rate
	Calcitonin (CT)	Regulates calcium metabolism; more active in children
Parathyroid Gland	Parathyroid hormone (PH)	Increases blood calcium levels through action on bone, kidneys and intestine
Thymus	Thymosin	Develops T lymphocytes
Pancreas (will be discussed in Chapter 5)	Insulin	Is required to store energy; regulates blood sugar levels; influenced by body weight
	Glucagon	Increases blood sugar levels
Adrenal Glands	Epinephrine	A component of the fight-or-flight response. Increases heart rate, facilitates blood flow to the muscles and brain, and helps with conversion of glycogen to glucose in the liver
	Norepinephrine	Has strong vasoconstrictive effects, increasing heart rate and blood pressure

GLAND	HORMONE	ACTION
Adrenal Glands (continued)	Hydrocortisone	Commonly known as cortisol; regulates how the body converts fats, proteins and carbohydrates into energy; helps regulate blood pressure and cardiovascular function
	Corticosterone	Works with hydrocortisone to regulate immune response and suppress inflammatory reactions
	Aldosterone	Maintains the right balance of salt and water while helping control blood pressure
	Dehydroepiandrosterone (DHEA)	Serves as a precursor to male and female sex hormones (androgens and estrogens); improves memory, mood, immune system and longevity
Ovaries	Estrogen	Manages reproductive maturation, regulation of menstrual cycles; decreases appetite
	Progesterone	Manages the regulation of menstrual cycles; serves as the hormone of gestation (pregnancy); increases appetite in the presence of estrogen
	Testosterone	Affects libido, energy and muscle mass; can increase appetite in the presence of estrogen

As you can see, our hormones can affect our emotions, weight and body composition. Cultivating your endocrine health, combined with proper nutrition and diet, can improve your appetite, reduce insomnia, relieve depression symptoms, improve circulation, boost your energy and relieve muscle pain. It takes putting all of the pieces of the puzzle together to successfully optimize your health. Honoring the mind-body-spirit connection is imperative for a woman to find hormonal health.

Fortunately, the *Eat Like a Woman* 3-step plan supports hormonal health! Each step will give you tools to keep those hormones in balance on a day-to-day basis. Each meal and snack can determine which energy sources you are going to use for the next four to six hours, and what you eat can control your hormone responses.

Chapter 3
Neurotransmitters:
Emotional Chemistry

Once again, let's start with a brief quiz.

YES	NO	SYMPTOM
		Do you feel insecure?
		Do you have problems sleeping?
		Do you feel anxiety for no reason?
		Do you have low self-esteem?
		Do you crave carbohydrates, alcohol, nicotine or drugs to calm yourself?
		Do you have difficulty concentrating?
		Do you have a low libido?
		Do you get panic attacks?
		Do you get aggressive for no reason?
		Do you have digestive problems?
		Do you have dry mouth?

continued on page 46

YES	NO	SYMPTOM
		Do you have a difficult time relaxing?
		Are you having memory problems?
		Do you feel worthless?
		Are you obsessive-compulsive?
		Are you suffering from an eating disorder?
		Do you feel depressed?

If you answered yes to any of these questions, you may have a neurotransmitter imbalance.

Neurotransmitters: The Spark That Connects Body and Brain

Just as glands secrete different types of hormones directly into the bloodstream to regulate the body, neurotransmitters are chemicals that serve as messengers between the brain and organs. These chemicals are released from a nerve cell that transmits an impulse to another nerve, muscle, organ or other tissue. Scientists do not yet know exactly how many neurotransmitters exist, but more than 100 chemical messengers have been identified! Research is only beginning to reveal the vast sex differences in neurotransmitters.

So what are some of the differences between hormones and neurotransmitters?

- Hormones are produced by an endocrine gland, and neurotransmitters are produced at nerve terminals when triggered by an electrical impulse.

- Hormones are secreted directly into the bloodstream, and neurotransmitters are secreted at nerve synapses.

- Hormones can be synthesized—for example, when a manufacturer makes hormone replacement therapy or thyroid replacement—but it is impossible to make neurotransmitters. They are made only inside the body.

Neurotransmitters play a major role in everyday life and functioning. These chemical messengers are molecular substances that can affect mood, appetite, sleep, heart rate, focus, metabolism and weight, temperature, and many other psychological and physical occurrences. Without neurotransmitters, your brain would not tell your heart to beat, lungs to breath, eyes to blink or stomach to digest. Depression and anxiety result from neurochemical imbalances. In fact, 1 in 10 Americans reports that they suffer from depression, the result of neurotransmitter imbalance.

How do neurotransmitters become imbalanced?

⬥ Chronic stress

⬥ Poor dietary habits (diets low in dietary protein, poor carbohydrate choices and low in omega-3 fats)

⬥ Environmental toxins: heavy metals, pesticides, bisphenol A (BPA), cleaning solvents, nicotine, alcohol, monosodium glutamate (MSG)

⬥ Medications: diet pills, stimulants, recreational drugs

⬥ Genetics

⬥ Sleep deprivation

⬥ Lack of good-quality sleep

⬥ Hormone imbalance

⬥ Excessive alcohol and caffeine usage

Women are twice as likely to suffer from depression and anxiety than men.

When your neurotransmitters are out of balance, you may experience the symptoms described in the quiz at the beginning of this chapter, as well as the following:

⬥ Weight problems

⬥ Depression

⬥ Fatigue

⬥ Migraines

⬥ Attention deficit disorder (ADD) or attention deficit hyperactivity disorder (ADHD)

⬥ Anxiety

⬥ Obsessive-compulsive disorder (OCD)

⬥ Behavioral issues

What you eat can influence your neurotransmitter levels, affecting your emotional health, which, in turn, fuels healthy food choices.

How Neurotransmitters Balance the Brain and Body

There are two kinds of neurotransmitters: inhibitory and excitatory.

As their name implies, **inhibitory** neurotransmitters tend to calm cells down. They help to control muscle activity and an important part of the visual system. Inhibitory neurotransmitters also calm the brain, induce sleep and help you relax. They balance mood and are easily depleted when the excitatory neurotransmitters are overactive. Gamma aminobutyric acid (GABA) and serotonin are two primary inhibitory neurotransmitters.

GABA is distributed throughout the central nervous system and is referred to as "nature's Valium-like substance." GABA gives you a calming feeling, increasing sleepiness and decreasing anxiety as well as muscle tension. Deficiency may cause extreme anxiety, panic, tenseness, insecurity, sleeplessness and even seizures. You may also have difficulty concentrating and suffer from constipation and eating disorders. Many compensate with Valium, alcohol, marijuana and sugar, hoping to find balance. The effects of having too much GABA can cause excess sleepiness and drowsiness.

As described in Chapter 2, serotonin is our feel-happy neurotransmitter. Serotonin is produced in the brain from the amino acid tryptophan and has to be balanced with melatonin. Serotonin affects our cravings, obsessive behavior, appetite, tranquility and peace of mind. It constricts blood vessels and brings on sleep. Serotonin also increases self-confidence, leads to a good mood and maintains body temperature while decreasing pain. Low serotonin levels are associated with decreased immune system function, and a deficiency may cause depression, mood disorders, insomnia, restlessness, dizziness, hypertension, obsessive-compulsive disorder, and anxiety, all of which increase cravings for alcohol, sugar, chocolate, tobacco and marijuana. There has been a whopping 400 percent increase in the prescribing of antidepressants since 1988, and antidepressants are the most commonly prescribed drug category in women aged 20 to 59 years. It is not surprising that women are two to three times more likely to develop depression, because females produce much less serotonin than males. People who have low serotonin tend to be stress eaters and have cravings for sweets and high-glycemic carbohydrates (desserts, French fries, chips, white bread and candy, such as jelly beans).

Studies have shown that women on a high-protein and low-carbohydrate diet are more prone to low serotonin levels. If you are serotonin depleted, this could cause initial weight gain while dieting and also increase cravings, mood disturbances and increase premenstrual syndrome (PMS).

Too much serotonin, however, may cause nausea and diarrhea, and if you abuse stimulant medications or caffeine in your daily regimen, it can cause a depletion of serotonin over time.

Serotonin also plays an important role in breastfeeding because it regulates milk production in the breast. Currently, research is being conducted on the belief that low serotonin levels may be the primary culprit for low breast milk production in nursing mothers.

The neurotransmitter systems involved with depression—serotonin, norepinephrine, dopamine, GABA and glutamate—all have receptors for estrogen and can be affected by the action of estrogen. It is no surprise so many women suffer from depression.

Excitatory neurotransmitters make cells more excitable, govern muscle contractions and cause glands to secrete hormones. Excitatory neurotransmitters stimulate the brain, so you feel energized, motivated and have clear focus.

One excitatory neurotransmitter is norepinephrine, which increases arousal, mental focus, alertness, learning, memory and mood regulation. Low levels of norepinephrine are associated with low energy, decreased focus and sleep cycle problems. A deficiency may cause depression and anxiety, possibly increasing a craving for alcohol, sugar, tobacco, caffeine and other substances, such as cocaine and marijuana. An excess of norepinephrine can fuel fear and anxiety, as may be the case for people who suffer from anxiety disorders.

Norepinephrine helps to make epinephrine as well. Epinephrine creates physical and emotional pain relief, pleasure, good feelings, euphoria and a sense of well-being. It also affects the metabolism of glucose and energy release during exercise, and it regulates your heart rate and blood pressure. Long-term stress or insomnia can cause epinephrine levels to be depleted. A deficiency may cause hypersensitivity to emotional and physical pain; inability to feel pleasure; a feeling of incompleteness; and cravings for alcohol, sugar, chocolate, heroin or marijuana.

There are some neurotransmitters that are both **inhibitory and excitatory,** such as acetylcholine (ACh) and dopamine. ACh was the first neurotransmitter to be identified in 1914. It is distributed throughout the central nervous system, where it is involved with arousal, learning, attention, memory, motivation and movement. In cardiac tissue, ACh neurotransmission has an inhibitory effect, which lowers heart rate. ACh also behaves as an excitatory neurotransmitter. A deficiency can cause Alzheimer's disease, dry mouth, inflammatory disorders, mood swings, and attention or memory problems. Too much ACh can cause violent muscle contractions.

Dopamine is the neurotransmitter that helps us focus and is responsible for emotional arousal and reward sensations. It is involved in a wide variety of behaviors such as setting goals, increasing pleasure, feelings of comfort, learning ability and being alert, and decreasing hunger. When dopamine is either elevated or low, we can have focus issues, such as not remembering where we put our keys, forgetting what a paragraph said when we just finished reading it, daydreaming, inability to handle stress, feeling worthless, mood swings and not being able to stay on task.

Dopamine is also responsible for our drive to get things done, or our motivation. A deficiency may cause depression, cravings for comfort or pleasure from substances (alcohol, caffeine, sugar, tobacco), schizophrenia and Parkinson's disease. Dopamine is naturally released before we wake up so we feel ready to wake up. It reduces with age and can be depleted by abusing drugs such as marijuana, speed, crack and cocaine.

The Brain-Gut Connection

There is a network of neurons lining our guts that is so extensive some scientists have nicknamed it our "second brain," despite the fact the gut is not the seat of any conscious thoughts or decision-making. The major neurotransmitters, a couple dozen small brain proteins called neuropeptides (those fabulous emotion-body connecters discussed in Chapter 2) and the major cells of the immune system, are also in the gut. In fact, almost 90 percent of the human body's total serotonin is found in specialized cells in our guts, not in our brain.

This isn't surprising if you consider that the gut and brain develop in an embryo from the same piece of tissue. The tissue eventually divides during development, one part going to the brain, the other to the gut. The body is an incredible creation!

The gut and brain are tied together by the vagus nerve, which starts in the brain and connects in the abdomen. When the brain senses a frightening situation, it releases stress hormones. Fear causes the vagus nerve to stimulate serotonin circuits in the gut. Once stimulated, the gut goes into higher gear and diarrhea can result.

The vagus nerve also regulates the heartbeat, and if you are stressed it can cause atypical heart pain. Additionally, the vagus nerve regulates the chemical levels in the digestive system so our daily nutritional intake can have a big effect on how we feel via our "second brain."

NEUROTRANSMITTER SUMMARY

Gamma aminobutyric acid (GABA)	Turns your brain off so you can relax; regulates awareness, movement and mood
Serotonin	Regulates mood, anxiety, appetite and sleep cycle; too little can make you crave carbs and have bad PMS
Acetylcholine (ACh)	Enhances memory and alertness
Dopamine	Creates feelings of motivation, focus and drive, as well as pleasure and enjoyment of food; an imbalance can be responsible for addictive disorders
Norepinephrine	Creates feelings of alertness, concentration and focus; lifts mood; raises blood pressure; can increase anxiety and affect metabolism
Epinephrine	Creates energy and focus; helps you cope with stress

The body is a beautifully designed machine. With adequate protein, healthy carbohydrates and fats, daily exercise, and awareness of the toxins in our world, we can manage neurotransmitter health.

How Hormones and Neurotransmitters Interact

We have gone on an incredible journey through our endocrine system and entered the fascinating world of neurotransmitters. Now let's look at how they dance together.

Hormonal changes can affect your neurotransmitters, and that has a direct response on how you feel, and that can affect lifestyle choices. For example, the relationship between estrogen and progesterone is delicate and can affect serotonin levels. When estrogen and progesterone levels change during the menstrual cycle or fluctuate during the menopausal years, you can experience moodiness, weight gain, PMS, menstrual headaches, decreased libido, hot flashes, vaginal dryness, difficulty sleeping and skin problems, all affecting serotonin, causing mild depression or the blues, and increasing the urge to crave sweets or carb-filled treats. Or when testosterone levels decrease naturally with age, childbirth and at menopause, dopamine is affected, so you feel like you have zero drive or can't motivate yourself. Additionally, declining testosterone can decrease your libido and muscle mass, as well as leave you feeling fatigued.

Just to make matters more complicated, lifestyle habits can affect your hormones, thereby affecting your neurotransmitters. For example, when you experience chronic levels of stress, it triggers surging cortisol, causing weight gain, cravings, insomnia, heart palpitations and even diabetes! Then, this vicious cycle can eventually affect serotonin levels and your thyroid, and a new set of problems pop up. The thyroid regulates your metabolism, and when those levels decline, it becomes difficult to manage a healthy weight, your nails may become brittle, cholesterol levels can change and you may have heavy periods; it can also make it difficult to get pregnant. Once this happens, serotonin levels decline, so you may feel depressed, moody and have a difficult time sleeping.

Wow! This is no simple fox trot—it's the quick-step in triple time! Lifestyle, hormones and neurotransmitters are all interrelated. When one fails to operate properly, the entire house of cards can fall.

Finding the Right Balance

As women, our bodies are in a constant state of change, and finding balance is critical so you feel good. Your lifestyle habits can alter your health. This is why it is so important to eat like a woman!

Eating and living healthy is important for both sexes, but it is especially critical for women. The complexity of our hormones—managing monthly periods, pregnancy, lactation and the major life stage changes—affects our neurotransmitters and how we feel. Our life experience as physical and spiritual beings is directly influenced by our daily choices.

While writing this chapter, I had a huge personal revelation about how my hormones, neurotransmitters and quality of life are all tied together. At the beginning of the hormone chapter,

I wrote about my terrible teenage years. I suffered from heavy periods, PMS, addiction to sweets, allergies and irritability. To continue that story, when I was in my 20s, a doctor discovered that I had a severe case of endometriosis, uterine fibroids and two huge ovarian cysts the size of oranges. And to top off the not-so-good news list, I was borderline hypoglycemic and had sleep issues. Today, I can recognize that my symptoms and conditions are the result of a complex interaction between my hormones and neurotransmitters at the different stages of my life.

The body is truly a sophisticated orchestration; without the proper arrangement, it would just be noise. One out-of-whack hormone can affect other hormones and neurotransmitters, and this is what happened with me.

Considering what we have discussed thus far, it does not seem too far-fetched that when the adrenals are stressed, the increased need to produce cortisol depletes the progesterone levels used in making cortisol. As more progesterone is diverted to make cortisol, less is available to balance the estrogen. When I had my hormone levels checked in my 20s, the estrogen-progesterone ratio was off balance, so I was on an estrogen-dominated runaway train.

My doctor surgically removed the ovarian cysts, endometrial tissue and fibroids—an eight-hour surgery—and put me on birth control pills to balance my out-of-whack hormones. That was 35 years ago, and I was lucky to have had an incredible doctor, Dr. Josephine Hall, who was an expert on women's health. In those days, most women in my situation got a full hysterectomy; I happily still have all of my organs.

Sadly, though, when I got off birth control pills at age 46 to find out if I was still "fertile," I slammed into menopause. All my previous symptoms from my teenage years resurfaced. It was a time of great struggle physically and emotionally. I have lived on a hormonal roller coaster and for much of my adult life required hormone therapy.

Could my situation have been managed with proper nutrition, exercise, stress management and sleep? My mother and her mother also suffered from the same calamities, so they were undoubtedly genetic. Unaware in my 20s and 30s of how to use nutrition to find hormonal balance, I never had the opportunity to try lifestyle changes before resorting to medications.

I invite you to note any hormone and neurotransmitter imbalances. Do the pieces of your health concerns start to make sense? Struggling with weight? Sleep issues? Irregular periods? Hot flashes? Depression? Visit an endocrinologist or women's health expert and discuss your symptoms. Collecting evidence so you can properly manage your health and weight with your practitioner is an important step to living empowered.

Neurotransmitter health supports good moods, self-confidence, energy, motivation and relaxation. Eat like a woman, and you will be able to nourish this sophisticated system—and you will be acknowledging that you are worth it. I wish I had this knowledge 35 years ago, but it is never too late to eat like a woman!

Chapter 4
Your Digestive System:
A Winding Road to Health

Women's digestive systems are so different from men's that I am shocked and angry that popular best-selling diet books have not created programs that embrace these differences. Yo-yo dieting is proof that these popular diet programs have not met our needs as women! Both sexes have the same digestive "parts," but how they function is different.

How Is Your Digestive System Different from a Man's?

Let's look at the many ways in which a woman's digestive system differs from a man's:

1. How you taste food is different. Women are more likely than men to be "supertasters." During pregnancy women have an increased sensitivity to bitter food due to changes in the hormone progesterone. This functions as a poison detector so a woman can protect herself and the fetus. There are different taste sensitivities to bitter foods depending on changes in hormones during the menstrual cycle. When a woman reaches menopause, this ability diminishes.

2. The esophagus, small intestine, colon and rectum of a woman are more sensitive than a man's. Women are at greater risk than men for developing irritable bowel syndrome (IBS), and women experience IBS symptoms at a more frequent rate during menstruation than at other times of their cycle. This may be due to hormonal changes that make controlling IBS symptoms more difficult for women. IBS causes, on average, 6.5 days of missed work per year for women. An estimated 30 million Americans suffer from IBS, approximately 70 percent of them are women. Reproductive hormones may be an influence

in this gender gap. Menstruation has been shown to aggravate the symptoms of IBS, and women with IBS are more likely to suffer from premenstrual syndrome and painful periods. The effects of estrogen and progesterone on IBS are still being researched, but the menstrual cycle seems to affect women suffering from IBS.

> The digestive system is all the organs and glands associated with the ingestion and digestion of food.

3. Your esophagus is shorter than a man's regardless of your height. A shorter length of the abdominal esophagus has shown a greater risk of esophageal irritation with acid reflux.

4. The muscles that prevent the backflow of food and stomach acid into the esophagus and windpipe are stronger and more efficient in women. This difference can increase a woman's protection against esophageal damage caused by heartburn and acid reflux. Therefore, males are more likely to have damage to the esophagus due to acid reflux. This damage can lead to abnormal cells in the esophagus (called Barrett's esophagus) that are precursors to esophageal cancer.

5. A woman secretes less stomach acid than a man, which may reduce her risk of developing acid-related ulcers.

6. Food can take longer to pass through the digestive system of women compared with that of men, increasing incidences of nausea and bloating.

7. A woman's large intestine empties more slowly than a man's, increasing her risk of constipation. This difference disappears after menopause.

8. A woman's colon is longer and has more twists and turns than a man's because the colon must navigate around the uterus and ovaries. This can also contribute to constipation.

9. The hormones progesterone and estrogen can make a woman's gallbladder empty more slowly than a man's and increase the amount of cholesterol in her gallbladder, doubling her risk of developing gallstones.

10. The composition of bile, which is made in the liver and stored in the gallbladder, is different between the sexes: some of the breakdown products of bile increase women's risk for colon cancer and may also explain the higher incidence of inflammatory diseases of the intestine in females, including ulcerative colitis and Crohn's disease.

11. A woman has less intestinal enzyme activity that breaks down medications in the small intestine and liver, so she tolerates various medications differently than a man. Women are 50 to 75 percent more likely than men to experience an adverse drug reaction.

12. Hormones produced during pregnancy can affect a woman who has been diagnosed with inflammatory bowel disease (Crohn's disease or ulcerative colitis), possibly making the problem get better or get worse. Hormones can also increase a pregnant woman's experiences of nausea and heartburn.

13. For women, colon cancer (the third most frequent type of cancer for American women) may be associated with breast cancer and never giving birth to children. Related to this, women have an increased incidence of right-sided colon cancer, which is why women need a full colonoscopy for cancer screening because a flexible sigmoidoscopy will miss right-sided cancers. (Flexible sigmoidoscopy is like a "mini-colonoscopy" but only evaluates the left side of the colon.)

14. Women are more likely than men to feel overly full after eating and have more problems with bloating and gas immediately following a meal.

15. Pancreatic cancer occurs three times more frequently in men than in women. Research is ongoing to determine if estrogen and progesterone protect women from pancreatic cancer.

16. Women absorb and metabolize alcohol differently than men. Women have less body water than men of similar body weight, causing women to achieve higher concentrations of alcohol in the blood after drinking equivalent amounts of alcohol. Women also have smaller quantities of the enzyme dehydrogenase, which breaks down alcohol in the stomach. A woman will absorb about 30 percent more alcohol into her bloodstream than a man of the same weight who has consumed an equal amount of alcohol. Women also appear to eliminate alcohol from the blood faster than men. This finding may be explained by women's higher liver volume per unit of lean body mass, because alcohol is metabolized almost entirely in the liver.

These are some pretty overwhelming physical and hormonal differences! Yet the science of studying the effects of biological sex on gastrointestinal function and on sex-specific nutritional requirements is still in its infancy.

Before moving forward to discover how we can take this fascinating new information and apply it to our lives, let's look at the basic operations of our digestive system.

25 Feet to Health

The main mission of the digestive system is to break down foods into nutrients in preparation for absorption. The gastrointestinal (GI) tract is a flexible tube of approximately 25 feet in length that extends from the mouth, through the esophagus, stomach, small intestine, large intestine and rectum, to the anus. It is an incredible design—the human body surrounds the GI tract for nourishment. It's like the kitchen in your home: everyone hangs out in the kitchen waiting to be fed.

While we are on the subject of food, let's follow the journey of food through the GI tract.

The Mouth

Most women are "supertasters" and have a great sense of smell. We may have good feelings associated with our food because we have a deeper limbic (emotional) system in the brain (see Chapter 2).

When you begin to chew, saliva, containing a starch-digesting enzyme, moistens the food and starts the digestion process. Chewing exposes saliva to the food for a longer period of time, allowing proper lubrication before swallowing. It also activates a signal to the GI system, triggering it to begin the entire digestive process. It's also best to keep chewing until you can no longer tell what kind of food you are eating from the texture of the food in your mouth (not the flavor). There is no magic number for the amount of times you should chew; it's all about texture.

Women have lower salivary rates, particularly during the menstrual period and post menopause, that can contribute to bad breath. The salivary flow is greater in males because they have a larger salivary gland.

The Stomach

You then swallow the chewed-up bits, moving them from your mouth through the esophagus to your stomach for the next phase of digestion that will churn, mix and grind the food to a liquid. The food gets mixed together and broken down into smaller pieces. Carbohydrate digestion continues until the mashed food has been mixed with the gastric juices; the stomach acid of the gastric juices inactivates the salivary enzyme, and carbohydrate digestion ends.

Estrogen can affect the amount of gastric acid secretion, leading to lower levels of this acid in women than in men.

Proteins begin to uncoil when they mix with the gastric acid, making them available to the gastric protease enzymes that begin to digest proteins. Fat forms a separate layer on the top of a watery mixture. It takes a longer time for food to empty from the stomach and enter the small intestines for reproductive women during certain times of their cycle; even non-menstruating females take a third longer for solids and twice as long for liquids when compared to men. More women suffer from bloating and belching in part due to the effect of progesterone on the gut than men.

The digestive system has two main hormones that control hunger and appetite. When your stomach is empty, it sends out a hormone called ghrelin, increasing your appetite. After you have eaten, the stomach secretes another hormone called leptin, telling your brain that you are full. Women produce more leptin because we have more fat, and leptin is produced by fat cells.

Two factors affect leptin's process: lack of sleep and high-fructose corn syrup (HFCS). When you don't get enough sleep, your body produces more ghrelin, the "I'm hungry" hormone, and less leptin, the "I'm full" hormone. HFCS found in sodas and other sweet processed foods inhibits leptin secretion. Have you ever wondered why you crave another soda after the first? That HFCS blocks the message that your stomach is full.

The Pancreas: Sugar Beware

The pancreas is located across the back of the upper abdomen, behind the stomach. It has many functions, playing a role in digestion as well as hormone production. Functions of the pancreas are as follows:

- The pancreas produces enzymes that break down food and hormones that help metabolize carbohydrates.
- It secretes hormones that affect the level of sugar in the blood.
- The pancreas completes the job of breaking down protein, carbohydrates and fats using its own digestive juices combined with juices from the intestines.
- It produces chemicals that neutralize stomach acids that pass from the stomach into the small intestine by using substances in pancreatic juices.
- It contains the islets of Langerhans, which are tiny groups of specialized cells that are scattered throughout the pancreas. These hormone-secreting cells produce glucagon and insulin, which are secreted directly into the bloodstream. Insulin and glucagon work together to maintain a steady level of glucose, or sugar, in the blood and to keep the body supplied with fuel to produce and maintain stores of energy. Glucagon raises the level of glucose (sugar) in the blood, and it increases with age.

Insulin stimulates cells to use glucose and is required to store energy and synthesize proteins from amino acids. It is produced after meals and when blood sugar is elevated. If insulin levels are low, you will feel tired because your cells do not receive enough glucose. When levels are high, insulin receptors shut down and you store excess glucose as body fat. Eating excess high-glycemic carbohydrates and processed foods raises insulin levels, burning out our receptor sites and making it hard for us to stop our cravings for sweets. This can lead to obesity and adult-onset diabetes, which is an imbalance of blood sugar levels, the major disorder of the pancreas.

Symptoms of low blood sugar include anxiety, sweating, increased heart rate, weakness, hunger and light-headedness. Dr. Jenkins says that "clinically it is very common for women, more than men, to report low blood sugar, then search out a sweet carb treat to solve the problem, only to continue on the blood sugar roller coaster."

The *Eat Like a Woman* program is designed to promote blood sugar balance with five to six small meals a day that consist of protein and a healthy carbohydrate, such as turkey and veggies or low-fat string cheese and fruit.

The Small Intestine

The next stop is the small intestine, which is approximately 20 feet long. Here, digestion continues, nutrients begin to be absorbed and water enters the body via blood and the lymph. Sugars require little digestion and begin to traverse the intestinal cells immediately on contact.

Starch digestion picks up when the pancreas sends pancreatic enzymes to the small intestine via the pancreatic duct and begins absorbing starches into the body. Small fragments of protein are now processed and absorbed through the cells of the small intestinal wall.

Fats are emulsified with the watery digestive fluids by bile. Now the fat can be absorbed through the cells of the small intestinal wall and into the lymph.

Vitamins A, D, E and K are fat soluble and travel through the lymphatic system of the small intestines and into the general blood circulation within the body. These fat-soluble vitamins, especially vitamins A and E, are then stored in body tissues. They can build up to toxic levels and become dangerous, so it is important to pay attention to the amount you are taking in supplements.

Vitamins B and C are water soluble. They enter the body and are put to work immediately, and any excess is eliminated from the body via the urine. Have you ever noticed that your urine is bright yellow after taking a vitamin—yep, it's those water-soluble vitamins, in and out!

Next, the vitamins and minerals are absorbed. First the vitamins that dissolve in water, then the vitamins that are dissolved in fat.

We digest carbohydrates first, then protein and finally fat. As mentioned previously, women take an hour longer than men to empty our stomachs so that our bodies can grab every morsel of the carbohydrates and calories. This phenomenon partly explains the often-expressed frustration that, "Men lose weight easier than women."

Knowing this, it seems logical to assume if we just ate protein first, then carbs, then fats, we would lose weight easier. This philosophy, in fact, opened the door to many diet programs being developed that combined certain foods. These programs are based on the theory that different food groups are digested optimally when eaten in certain combinations, such as eating fruits alone or eating protein and starches at separate meals. It's also been suggested that poor digestion from improper food combinations will weaken you and stress your immune system. In reality, these ideas make for excellent book sales, but do not optimize your health.

The food-combining theory is a myth. According to the Academy of Nutrition and Dietetics,

> *There is no evidence that combining certain foods or eating foods at specific times of day will help with weight loss. Eating the 'wrong' combinations of food doesn't cause them to turn to fat immediately or to produce toxins in your intestines, as some plans claim.*

The food-combining theory represents faulty logic and a huge underrepresentation of the body's capabilities.

The Large Intestine

Our food journey continues, moving now from the small intestine to the large intestine. The large intestine passes waste (fiber, bacteria and unabsorbed nutrients) along with water to the rectum.

The body contains trillions of bacteria, both good and bad. Most live in our gut, but they also colonize in other areas, including the large intestine. The good bacteria help digest food, protect us from infection, and produce vitamins. A probiotic (taken orally in supplement or liquid form) adds good bacteria and can alleviate diarrhea, constipation, inflammatory bowel disease, vaginal infections, ulcers, allergies and lactose intolerance, and help enhance immune function.

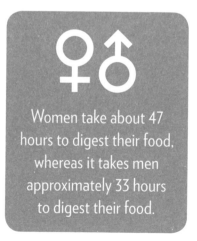

Women take about 47 hours to digest their food, whereas it takes men approximately 33 hours to digest their food.

Eating yogurt daily is also a great way to create balance and improve digestion. Vitamins produced by the live cultures in yogurt include biotin, folate, pantothenic acid, riboflavin, thiamin, vitamin B_6, vitamin B_{12} and vitamin K.

Some fibers are partly digested by the bacteria living in the large intestine, and some of these products are absorbed. Most fibers pass through the large intestine and are excreted as feces; some fat, cholesterol, and minerals bind to fiber and are also excreted. The digestive system eliminates all indigestible substances as stool.

Caring for Your Digestive System

The 25-foot food journey is simple yet complex, from top to bottom (no pun intended)—foods must be broken down into small particles and suspended in enough liquid so that every particle is accessible to nourish our body. You'll recall that hormones and neurotransmitters that affect blood sugar, appetite and bowel function are also produced in the digestive system. Clearly, the health of our endocrine system, neurotransmitters and digestive system are all connected.

The following list outlines some common GI problems that can result from imbalances in the digestive system, as well as strategies you can use to prevent or alleviate them:

STRATEGIES TO PREVENT OR ALLEVIATE COMMON GI PROBLEMS

SYMPTOM	ACTION
Diarrhea due to IBS	• Rest. • Drink fluids to replace losses. • Exercise regularly. • Respond promptly to the urge to go. • Avoid sensitizing foods. • Avoid stress.
Constipation	• Eat a high-fiber diet. • Drink plenty of fluids. • Exercise regularly. • Respond promptly to the urge to go. • Ensure adequate fiber intake.

SYMPTOM	ACTION
Belching	♦ Eat slowly. ♦ Chew thoroughly. ♦ Relax while eating.
Intestinal gas	♦ Eat bothersome food in moderation. ♦ Passing gas around 13–21 times per day is normal. However, eating excessive carbs can cause excessive gas. Carbs that can cause gas include the following: beans, broccoli, cauliflower, cabbage, brussels sprouts, onions, mushrooms, artichokes, asparagus, pears, apples, peaches, whole grains, sodas, apple juice, pear juice, milk, cheese, ice cream, yogurt, sugar-free candies and gums that contain sugar alcohols such as sorbitol, mannitol, and xylitol.
Heartburn	♦ Eat small meals. ♦ Drink liquids between meals. ♦ Sit up while eating. If you are bedbound, elevate your head when eating. ♦ Wait 3 hours after eating before lying down. ♦ Wait 2 hours after eating before exercising. ♦ Refrain from wearing tight-fitting clothes. ♦ Avoid foods, beverages and medications that aggravate your heartburn (some of your favorites, such as chocolate, fruit juice and mint, are common culprits). ♦ Refrain from smoking cigarettes or using tobacco products. ♦ Lose weight if you are overweight.

continued on page 62

SYMPTOM	ACTION
Ulcer	• Take medication as prescribed by your physician. • Avoid coffee, caffeine and alcoholic beverages. • Avoid foods that aggravate your ulcer. • Do not use anti-inflammatories, such as aspirin, ibuprofen and naproxen, without your doctors approval. • Refrain from smoking cigarettes.

Source: Understanding Nutrition *by Ellie Whitney and Sharon Rady Rolfes, 2011, Wadsworth, Cengage Learning.*

There are many things you can do to contribute to the health of your digestive system:

1. Get plenty of sleep. Adequate sleep allows for repair and maintenance of tissue and removal of wastes that might impair efficient functioning.

2. Stay active. Physical activity promotes healthy muscle tone to support your GI tract.

3. Maintain a positive outlook. A positive attitude influences the activity of regulatory nerves and hormones.

4. Make time to enjoy your meal. Mealtime should be relaxed.

5. Eat meals that promote optimal absorption of nutrients.

6. Enjoy a variety of foods.

7. Eat in moderation—neither too much nor too little of anything.

8. Enjoy a cup of yogurt daily. Many brands of yogurt have HFCS. Look at the ingredients, and buy plain, natural yogurt and sweeten with fruit. FAGE Total 2 percent is one of my favorites.

9. Eat fiber to keep food moving through the digestive tract.

10. Avoid foods with high levels of HFCS (sodas, most salad dressings, canned fruit, applesauce, cereal bars, frozen pizza).

You may note that these tips are similar to the tips for maintaining your endocrine system and neurotransmitter health. An amazing pattern is unfolding, and paying attention to it is a simple way to change your life by embracing the needs of a woman's body.

Step 1 of the *Eat Like a Woman* program, outlined in Chapter 7, will reveal an easy system to apply all this information to your daily life.

Chapter 5
The Secret Life of Your Fat Cells

> "I feel fat today."
>
> "Do I look fat in these jeans?"
>
> "I'm too fat to wear a swimsuit."
>
> "My cellulite makes my legs look fat."
>
> "I don't want to go to the gym because I am so fat."

How many times have you said or thought you were fat? Women of all sizes feel fat. I have been guilty of spending a portion of a girls' night out talking about weight—just lost some, up a few pounds, need to lose some more. Why are American women so obsessed with their weight?

One of my theories is that fashion today is more revealing, and looking like a normal, healthy woman isn't always possible when your tush is hanging out of a pair of short shorts, or when your tummy is pouring over the super-low hip-hugger jeans with a 2-inch zipper. Even 12-year-olds have a hard time looking and feeling good in these fashions!

The media and size-0-obsessed fashion industry use Photoshop software to modify most of the images we see. Being an American woman surrounded by these images of overly thin women can leave a normal, healthy woman with a poor self-image and low self-esteem. What the medical community says is a healthy weight is often considered fat by many women. We have been brainwashed to think a size 0, 2 or 4 is the norm.

For some cultures, a woman at a healthy weight represents fertility, wealth and health. But something has become warped in American culture over the past 100 years or so. At the turn of the 20th century in America, Lillian Russell was a 200-pound sex symbol. There were programs available to women at that time to help them increase their weight so they would look like Ms. Russell. Thinner women were regarded as unattractive and poor.

What happened in America to turn this attitude around? Historian Peter Stearns, Ph.D., at George Mason University claims obesity became strongly associated with the sin of gluttony and a sign of moral weakness during the late 19th and early 20th centuries with the influence of Protestant values. It may have been a response to the new abundance of food and increase in consumerism. Yet during World War I, with concerns about food storages, many popular magazines promoted the message that gaining weight was unpatriotic. By the 1950s, being fat was unpopular, and women started taking diet drugs and having surgery to stay thin.

In the 1960s, the media promoted beauty by using ultra-thin models like Twiggy, and a shapely beauty like Marilyn Monroe was out of fashion. Since that time, beauty has become more and more equated with unnatural thinness.

Women are not the only victims. Today men, too, feel pressure to be more trim and muscular. Physical appearance has become an American obsession. Being slim has become synonymous with being more attractive or smarter and more talented. Unjustly, many overweight people are stereotyped as gluttonous and lazy, resulting in discrimination at work and in social situations.

Unfortunately, women in the United States tend to be discontented with their bodies because of their weight. Between the two sexes, men are generally more satisfied with their bodies, heavy or not.

Surveys have revealed that girls as young as six years old are going on diets because they think they are fat, and by age nine, over half of all girls in America have already gone on a diet. It is no surprise that girls struggle with the natural transition into puberty when almost one-third of their adult weight is gained. Even after childbirth, women feel pressured to lose their baby weight and flatten their stomachs immediately. Celebrities go on crash diets to lose their baby weight and then publicly show the world their bodies once again returned to their pre-pregnancy state only two months later. Our society denies the natural, ever-changing function of a woman's body.

Combine the influence of the media using thin models with a multibillion-dollar beauty/fashion industry, and it is no surprise that women and men feel inadequate about their appearance. Even when a woman feels good about herself on the inside, being bombarded with images of overly thin young women can make it difficult for her to accept herself. Many struggle with eating disorders, including the models and actresses we try to imitate.

The companies and individuals producing extreme dieting programs, liposuction, anti-fat medications, spa body wraps and body shapewear garments are making a fortune off of our desire to be fat-free. Instead of celebrating health, so many women focus on unrealistic expectations for thinness, breeding insecurity and unhappiness.

This dysfunctional cycle has produced the exact opposite of people being thin. About two-thirds of Americans are overweight now. Second to smoking, obesity is the leading cause of preventable deaths. While this book was in production, the American Medical Association's House of Delegates approved a resolution recognizing obesity as a disease that requires treatment and prevention efforts.

So what *is* contributing to obesity in the United States?

Genetics?	Fast food?	Socioeconomic status?
Toxins?	Super-sized portions?	Psychological issues?
Sugar?	Cultural expectations?	Metabolic problems?
Wheat?	Behavior?	

Perhaps some or all of these factors contribute to obesity, and there are some factors we have little control over. We do, however, have power over our expectations, attitudes and lifestyle choices. Now is the time to focus on health and to celebrate that we are all different.

Women come in all shapes and sizes, and different people are healthy at different weights. For a woman with a large frame, being a size 4 is impossible, but at a size 12 she is fit and healthy. Does that make this woman unattractive? No! Many women struggle with their size because the media shows young female celebrities wearing a size 0 or 2, yet today the average American woman is 5'4", has a waist size of 34 inches to 35 inches, and weighs between 140 and 150 pounds, with a dress size of 12 to 14.

Additionally, a woman's weight can "naturally" fluctuate for many reasons: stress, pregnancy, premenstrual syndrome (PMS), menopause, age, disease, lack of sleep and unhappiness. We must start seeing a woman's healthy weight as attractive, regardless of the size of her clothes. For some women, having a small frame and being naturally thin is healthy; for others, a large frame and curvy body is healthy. Coming to Twiggy's defense, she may have naturally been a very thin person and filled out naturally as she aged, as we all do. But the media portrayed her as the ideal beauty, and that's where the trouble began. We must demand that the media represent women's bodies as attractive in all sizes. I no longer purchase magazines that use extremely thin models to represent women as a whole.

Are we naturally finding our healthy weight, going on diets in attempts to become a size 2, and then, in the process, actually gaining weight? Our toxic body culture is breeding low self-esteem, yo-yo dieting and poor health.

Why has women's health been marginalized, and how did our weight become a never-ending conversation? Even famous female politicians have their appearance scrutinized—she looks fat in this, or tired in that, or she had Botox. Does anyone ever notice if a suit makes their male counterparts look fat or if their haircut makes them look older? No!

If we can enjoy life as confident women focusing on health, rather than weight, and on our contributions to life rather than appearance, perhaps self-acceptance and self-esteem will rise in America.

Let's Get Real About Fat

There are many differences between a woman's body fat and a man's.

1. Women generally have a higher percentage of body fat than men. A healthy woman's body fat content is 20 to 25 percent versus 10 to 15 percent for a man.

2. Women are born with more fat cells. And the fat cells in a woman's body are five times larger than a man's, which means there is more room for storage.

3. Women require fewer daily calories per pound of body weight than men. If you eat as much as a man, even at comparable exercise levels, you will probably gain weight simply because women do not need as much fuel as men.

4. During puberty, a girl's fat increase almost doubles compared to that of boys. When a teenage girl reaches around 17 percent body fat, menarche occurs, with the average age between 12 and 13.5 years old.

5. By age 25, healthy-weight women have almost twice the body fat that healthy-weight men have.

6. Female hormones make it easier to convert fat into storage to support pregnancy and breastfeeding. Having an environment that can protect a fetus is important to both mother and child.

7. The Institute of Medicine recommends a weight gain of 15 pounds during pregnancy. Less than one-third of U.S. women honor this recommendation. Higher body mass index (BMI) during pregnancy is associated with increased risks for gestational diabetes, preeclampsia, gestational hypertension, prolonged labor, caesarean delivery and postpartum anemia.

8. As we age, women tend to gain about 10 percent fat and weight each decade during adulthood. Lack of physical activity along with a steady decline in metabolic rate is mostly to blame.

9. Blood flow and transport of fats to the lower body is greater in women compared to men. When you enjoy a yummy dessert and say, "It's going straight to my hips," you are correct. Those sweets are going right to your fat cells.

10. Women burn more fat for fuel than men after longer durations of exercise and men burn more carbohydrates.

11. Estrogen reduces a woman's ability to burn energy after eating, resulting in more fat being stored around the body. No doubt, this happens to prime a woman for childbearing.

12. Aging increases adiposity in both sexes, but a woman has a higher percent of body fat throughout her entire life span. Studies demonstrate that genetic factors account for up to 70 percent of BMI variance, and the genetic factor can be even greater for women. It may all sound depressing because women are built to store fat, but here is some good news. All women before menopause have less intra-abdominal adipose tissue, with fat being stored in the hips, thighs and tush area (pear shape) instead, making for a more favorable metabolic risk profile. Men with similar total body fat store it in the belly area (apple shape). This visceral fat is metabolically active tissue and is more toxic. However, this protection against visceral belly fat accumulation is lost when women enter menopause. This happened to me when I slammed into menopause. Fortunately, I figured out a system to save myself and started eating like a woman.

> The word *adipose* comes from the Latin *adeps* meaning "fat, grease or lard."

13. A study found a higher content of intramuscular triglycerides (fat stored directly within muscle fibers) in women. Many women spend hours doing cardio hoping to reduce fat, but they should also be pumping weights and resistance training. This combination will help achieve muscular tone by managing that fat located in the muscle fiber.

14. There are major sex differences in insulin sensitivity in adipose tissue, particularly in the belly, that are regulated by physiological levels of sex hormones. Women have a lower level of insulin resistance and diabetes risk than men despite similar or higher fat content.

15. Women store a greater percentage of dietary fatty acids in subcutaneous adipose tissue, located just beneath the skin, than men. That is why our skin looks bumpier than men's, even with toned muscles.

16. Women have different leptin levels than men. You'll recall that leptin is a hormone produced by the fat cells that controls appetite, energy and metabolic rate (see Chapter 3). Women have a higher level of the adipose tissue–derived hormone leptin because we naturally have more fat. In fact, a new study suggests that women who had higher levels of leptin had decreased symptoms of anxiety and depression. This is good news, but if someone is overweight, that person can become "leptin resistant." There is more fat making more leptin, but it is not working properly—instead of telling the brain you are full, you actually get hungrier. Therefore, this is a good reason to get those fat cells working properly and obtain a healthy weight.

17. Women have higher levels of adiponectin, a hormone derived from visceral fat that sensitizes the body to insulin, has anti-inflammatory properties, and plays a role in the metabolism of glucose and lipids. Adiponectin is the only hormone secreted by the fat cell that actually helps to prevent adverse conditions such as diabetes, cardiovascular disease, obesity, inflammation and metabolic syndrome (pre-diabetes). When levels of adiponectin decrease, visceral fat accumulation results. Obese women have a lower level of adiponectin.

With all these fat cell sex differences, it seems unthinkable that women and men would have the same response to the same diet. When it comes to fat cells, it may feel like having two X chromosomes is a disadvantage, but our fat cells actually give women an advantage. Women were designed to survive—you can use this advantage to lose and maintain your weight, reduce your risk of some diseases and manage a healthy weight without dieting. Sound good? Let's take a field trip through the fat cell factory so we can learn about how to take advantage of what it produces.

The Amazing Fat Cell

The fat cell has many wonderful purposes:

- It provides energy for the body.
- It stores excess calories for future use.
- It insulates your body, keeping you warm.
- It provides padding to protect internal organs and bones.
- It regulates bodily functions, including hormone production and thermogenesis (the production of heat).
- It contours the body—fat gives us our great "curves."
- It stores some vitamins.
- It helps the body use protein and carbohydrates.
- It is a major ingredient of brain tissue.
- It is a structural component of all cell membranes.

Fewer than 100 years ago, there were no one-stop shopping markets. Many had to milk a cow for a glass of milk, make a trip to the bakery for bread or go to the butcher for meat. Our bodies are designed to go extended periods of time between meals. Our ancestors of 40,000 years ago often went days without a proper meal, so in between meals, they needed a source of energy. That's where fat cells come in.

The fat cells oversee the body's energy and how it's used. Fat cell receptors control metabolism by instructing muscles to burn energy or by telling the liver when to store fuel supplies. They also discharge chemicals that stimulate appetite; change insulin levels; and affect the immune system, blood vessel constriction and reproduction. If a woman has less than 8 percent body fat, she may not be able to have her monthly period or conceive.

Fat cells are called adipose cells because they live in adipose tissue, also known as fatty tissue. The fat stored in adipose cells comes from dietary fats or is produced in the body.

Types of Body Fat

There are two types of fat in the body:

Essential fat is the type of fat needed for normal physiological and biological functioning. It is found in bone marrow, the brain, spinal cord, cell membranes, muscles, and other internal organs. Women also deposit essential fat in the breasts and the area surrounding the uterus. Women have 12 percent of their total body weight in essential fat compared to 3 percent for men. If essential fat drops below the critical level, normal functions may be impaired.

Nonessential fat, also known as storage fat or subcutaneous fat, is typically layered below the skin. It insulates the body to retain heat, pads the body against trauma, and provides energy during rest and exercise. Nonessential fat stored around the internal organs in the abdominal cavity is referred to as visceral fat—the unpopular belly fat.

A healthy range of body fat for women aged 34 to 55 years is 25 to 32 percent, with most of the fat being stored in the hips and buttocks area, and then shifting upward after menopause. For men of the same age group, it is 10 to 18 percent, with men carrying most of their fat in the belly area.

Types of Fat Cells

Those two types of body fat contain three types of fat cells:

White adipose tissue stores excess calories in the form of jiggly thighs and a jelly belly. It is important in energy metabolism, heat insulation and padding for internal organ protection. If we lived in a world with limited food resources, white fat cells could save our lives.

Brown adipose tissue releases stored energy as heat. Brown fat is needed for making heat by burning calories (thermogenesis), and it has the ability to burn high quantities of fat and sugar. Brown fat is found between the shoulders, and newborn babies have lots of it to keep warm. As we age, we have less brown fat. People who have more brown fat are less likely to be obese, but women tend to have more brown fat than men, which is great news! How do we make more brown fat?

Researchers at Sanford-Burnham Medical Research Institute recently discovered that shortages of the brain hormone orexin (responsible for wakefulness and appetite) in mice can generate weight loss by activating brown fat cells to release excess energy as heat instead of storing it. Orexin deficiency is associated with obesity.

Orexin-producing cells have recently been shown to be inhibited by glucose. Perhaps eating a high glycemic meal can reduce the fat burning effects of orexin? Stay tuned for new orexin research on humans, not just mice—I suspect it may hold an additional link to managing a healthy weight.

Beige adipose tissue was just recently discovered and is similar to brown fat cells in converting energy from food into heat. It can form from the undesirable white fat cells. Beige fat is scattered in pea-sized deposits beneath the skin near the collarbone and along the spine.

A research team led by Dr. Bruce Spiegelman from Harvard Medical School published a study revealing that during exercise, muscles release the hormone called irisin, which then converts ordinary white fat cells into beige ones—and those beige cells help the body burn more energy. The study was conducted on mice, but Dr. Spiegelman found that humans also have irisin. While not yet proven, it is very likely that irisin has similar effects in people.

The Life of a Fat Cell

We know women are born with more fat cells than men, but do we have the same number forever? We could, but most of us in the western world of the ever-expanding waistline do not.

Fat cell development is an easy process, and once you grow a new fat cell you will always have it. Fat cells are capable of increasing their size by 20-fold and their number by several thousand-fold. Yikes!

Adipose produces the satiety hormone, leptin, and the hormone adiponectin, which is involved in regulating glucose levels as well as fatty acid breakdown, so the fat cell is now considered an endocrine organ. Adipose plays a prominent role in energy metabolism. Fat cells have an enzyme called estrogen synthase (aromatase), which converts whatever male hormones (androgens) are in the vicinity into female hormones (estrogens). This phenomenon, which occurs in both men and women, means that the more fat tissue one has, the greater the estrogen influence in the body. This increased estrogen influence is problematic because it may increase the risk for breast and uterine cancer in women.

Here's how a fat cell grows and multiplies:

1. When energy intake exceeds expenditure, your fat cells increase in size. If you are not using fat for energy, it has to go somewhere, so it goes to the fat storage center.

2. When fat cells have enlarged because you are not using them for energy, and they get to their maximum size, they divide and increase in number again. This is called mitosis.

3. With weight loss, the size of the fat cells shrinks but not the number.

As you age and your metabolism slows down, the amount of fat in your body slowly increases. Women experience an even greater fat percentage increase than men do. Cells can direct the body to store additional fat even though eating habits are not increased dramatically. This explains the frustration women experience during menopause. Despite healthy eating habits and daily exercise, most women continue to add weight. For that reason, menopause can be challenging, because it takes greater effort to maintain the same weight as the reproductive years. But we can control the size of the fat cell.

We can't discuss fat without giving equal time to cellulite, that orange peel–look on the hips, tush and thighs. Cellulite is another word for fat, and it looks like cottage cheese—80 to 90 percent of post-pubertal females have cellulite. Cellulite got a bad rap in the '60s when it was referenced in *Vogue* magazine. Perhaps no one discussed it until our skirt hems got short enough to see that women have different-looking upper thighs than men.

This appearance is much more common in women than in men because of differences in the way fat, muscle and connective tissue are distributed in men's and women's skin. Women have cellulite because our collagen structure has the appearance of a picket fence, as opposed to a man's, which looks like a cross-linked fence holding the fat in better. Estrogen encourages fat, whereas testosterone breaks down fat.

> Green tea extract contains many compounds, including catechins, that have been shown to help burn off fat. Green tea also contains an amino acid called L-theanine that has a relaxing effect on the brain and body.

When fat cells increase in size, they can become visible through the skin, and as we get older and our skin becomes thinner, it is even more visible. You do not need to be overweight to have cellulite; some of the thinnest women have cellulite. Genetic predisposition may make you more prone to having cellulite.

Our present-day diet has probably been a cellulite culprit, as well as being less active with modern conveniences. There is no cream, pill or other gimmick that will get rid of cellulite, so don't waste your money. Once you begin the *Eat Like a Woman* program and find your healthy weight, those fat cells will shrink and cellulite will not look as bad.

The Fats in Food

Food contains three kinds of fats, all of which have a critical function in maintaining good health:

* Triglycerides, which make adipose tissue and are used for energy.
* Phospholipids, which transport hormones and fat-soluble vitamins (A, D, E and K) through your blood, flowing across cell membranes through a watery fluid.
* Sterols, which are a fat and alcohol compound with zero calories; vitamin D, testosterone and cholesterol are sterols.

As you will recall from the previous chapter, fats go through the same digestive process but are digested after carbohydrates and proteins. Fat is then used for storage or energy. However, the body prefers to grab glucose from carbs for energy, because it is easier and more efficient than burning fat.

How we feel about our fat and body shape can influence our emotional health, but many women struggle with self-image.

Women and Eating Disorders

In the United States, 20 million women and 10 million men suffer from a clinically significant eating disorder at some time in their life, including anorexia nervosa, bulimia nervosa, binge-eating disorder or an eating disorder not otherwise specified. Although there is no single known cause of eating disorders, culture, emotional disorders, a life change or stressful event, biology, family attitudes about appearance, and genetics may contribute. Eating disorders frequently develop during adolescence or early adulthood but can occur during childhood or later in adulthood. Eating disorders are serious emotional and physical problems that can have life-threatening consequences for women and men.

By age 6, girls especially start to express concerns about their own weight or shape, and 40 to 60 percent of elementary school girls, ages 6 to 12, are concerned about their weight or about becoming too fat.

According to the National Eating Disorders Association, the average American woman is 5'4" tall and weighs 140 pounds. The average American model is 5'11" tall and weighs 117 pounds. The average Miss America winner is 5'7" and weighs 121 pounds. The average BMI of Miss America winners has decreased from around 22 in the 1920s to 16.9 in the 2000s.

American society associates being "thin" with being hard-working, beautiful, strong and self-disciplined. On the other hand, being "fat" is associated with being lazy, ugly, weak and lacking willpower. Because of these harsh critiques, women are often dissatisfied with their bodies. As a result, they often feel great anxiety and pressure to achieve or maintain a weight that is not necessarily healthy.

Eating disorders are more than just a problem with food. Food is used to feel in control of other feelings that may seem overwhelming. For example, starving is a way for people with anorexia to feel more in control of their lives and to ease tension, anger and anxiety. Likewise, purging and other behaviors to prevent weight gain are ways for people with bulimia to feel that same level of control.

The National Eating Disorders Association has a list of doctors, nutritionists, counselors, and in-patient and/or out-patient facilities in your area.

Fat is a fact of life *and* necessary for life, but how much fat is healthy for you? Knowing your healthy weight can empower you to set realistic expectations so you can celebrate your shape as uniquely yours.

Chapter 6
What's Your Healthy Weight?

What's your healthy weight? This may be the most frustrating question for women today!

Perhaps you have been "classified" as overweight but have never felt healthier. Or you may be postmenopausal and trying to reach your college weight. You may be a teen struggling with obtaining the perfect shape as defined by fashion magazines. You may have just had a baby and feel embarrassed about your new voluptuousness.

As we've learned, for women up to the age of 45, a healthy range of body fat is 20 to 25 percent. The only variation is that it is acceptable for female athletes to have body fat percentages between 14 and 20 percent. A woman needs at least 12 percent body fat for her body to function normally with monthly periods and be fertile. Over the age of 45, the range for women extends up to 32 percent.

Body Fat Development During the Life Stages

Women tend to gain weight during puberty, post pregnancy and after menopause, making those life transitions especially challenging.

Here is a further breakdown of the body fat development during a woman's life stages:

Ages 16-18: Height growth stops; changes toward an adult body start.

Ages 19-23: Heading toward maturity, the female body shape emerges.

Ages 24-26: Transformation to an adult body completes.

continued on page 76

Ages 27–36: Extra subcutaneous fat is deposited in the body, gradually changing the body's shape. Those womanly curves!

Ages 37–39: Sudden weight gain begins. Body shape starts to drastically change.

Ages 40–46: The lower half of the body is visibly growing larger.

Ages 47+: Most women find their body shape gradually begins to change because visceral abdominal fat and subcutaneous abdominal fat ratios increase with age. Lower levels of estrogen and a slower metabolism due to natural aging can result in redistribution of body fat. Gradually the waist becomes larger, while the legs and arms become thinner.

A WOMAN'S BODY THROUGH DIFFERENT AGES

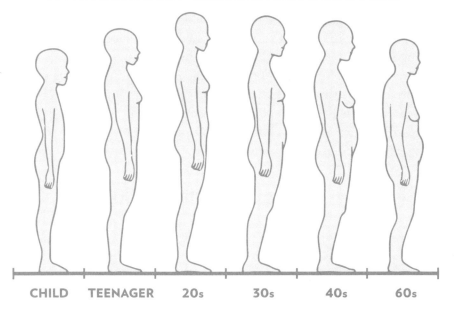

CHILD   TEENAGER   20s   30s   40s   60s

Child: Large head, curved back, slight protruding belly.
Teenager: Breasts start to grow and hips get rounded.
20s: Figure of a mature woman.

30s: Fat begins to saturate.
40s: Stomach grows and many women tend to worry about changes in their figures.
60s: The back becomes rounded, the frame curves.

Just as a woman's body shape changes with age throughout each life stage, so does her percentage of body fat.

BODY FAT PERCENTAGE STANDARDS FOR WOMEN RECOMMENDED BY AGE GROUP

	18 to 39	40 to 59	60+
Underfat	<20	<21	<22
Standard Minus	21-27	22-28	23-29
Standard Plus	28-34	29-35	30-36
Overfat	35-39	36-40	37-41
Obese	>40	>41	>42

Source: Gallagher D, et al. Am J Clin Nutr 2000;72:694-701. "Healthy percentage body fat ranges: an approach for developing guidelines based on body mass index."

How to Calculate Your Healthy Weight

There are many variables in determining a woman's "healthy" weight. Your weight is a reflection of your nutritional choices, daily physical activity, sleep habits, hormones, genetics, age, sex, family history, body composition and stress levels. Some of these factors we can manage; others are unchangeable. We can control what we eat, how much sleep we get, when we schedule physical activity and our stress levels.

The combination of your body type, frame size and body composition will determine your personal ideal weight. Because of these variables, we will use four formulas to calculate your healthy weight: 1) the body mass index (BMI) chart, 2) your waist-to-hip ratio, 3) your body fat and lean muscle mass, and 4) your frame size. These calculators/charts are available online at www.EatLikeAWoman.com. For those who want to crunch numbers, grab your pencil and let's begin.

> The *Eat Like a Woman* healthy weight philosophy is simple: Your best weight is the weight you can achieve and maintain while living the healthiest lifestyle possible and still be able to enjoy life!

What Is Your BMI?

The BMI chart below is the most common way health-care providers and others assess whether a person has too much body fat. This tool determines your health based on height and weight, but the BMI does not accurately represent the amount of body fat. After reading an entire chapter dedicated to a woman's fat cells, you know that determining your actual body fat percentage is an important part of the personalized "healthy weight" formula. That said, the BMI chart can be a useful tool for general groups, but on an individual basis, it is not accurate in accessing body fat. Someone who is very muscular might have a BMI over 25 but may not actually be overweight.

BODY MASS INDEX, A WOMAN'S BODY THROUGH DIFFERENT LIFE STAGES, BODY FAT PERCENTAGE STANDARDS BY AGE GROUP, FRAME SIZE RELATIVE TO WEIGHT

BMI	19	20	21	22	23	24	25	26	27	28	29	30	31	32	33	34	35
Height (inches)	Body Weight (pounds)																
58	91	96	100	105	110	115	119	124	129	134	138	143	148	153	158	162	167
59	94	99	104	109	114	119	124	128	133	138	143	148	153	158	163	168	173
60	97	102	107	112	118	123	128	133	138	143	148	153	158	163	168	174	179
61	100	106	111	116	122	127	132	137	143	148	153	158	164	169	174	180	185
62	104	109	115	120	126	131	136	142	147	153	158	164	169	175	180	186	191
63	107	113	118	124	130	135	141	146	152	158	163	169	175	180	186	191	197
64	110	116	122	128	134	140	145	151	157	163	169	174	180	186	192	197	204
65	114	120	126	132	138	144	150	156	162	168	174	180	186	192	198	204	210
66	118	124	130	136	142	148	155	161	167	173	179	186	192	198	204	210	216
67	121	127	134	140	146	153	159	166	172	178	185	191	198	204	211	217	223
68	125	131	138	144	151	158	164	171	177	184	190	197	203	210	216	223	230
69	128	135	142	149	155	162	169	176	182	189	196	203	209	216	223	230	236
70	132	139	146	153	160	167	174	181	188	195	202	209	216	222	229	236	243
71	136	143	150	157	165	172	179	186	193	200	208	215	222	229	236	243	250
72	140	147	154	162	169	177	184	191	199	206	213	221	228	235	242	250	258
73	144	151	159	166	174	182	189	197	204	212	219	227	235	242	250	257	265
74	148	155	163	171	179	186	194	202	210	218	225	233	241	249	256	264	272
75	152	160	168	176	184	192	200	208	216	224	232	240	248	256	264	272	279
76	156	164	172	180	189	197	205	213	221	230	238	246	254	263	271	279	287

Source: Centers for Disease Control and Prevention.

BMI Categories

Underweight = <18.5

Normal weight = 18.5–24.9

Overweight = 25–29.9

Obesity = BMI of 30 or greater

We are all different. We come in all shapes and sizes, and being in the BMI "overweight" category may not be as bad as you think. Recently, the *Journal of the American Medical Association* published a report conducted on nearly three million people by the Centers for Disease Control and Prevention and found that those with a BMI in the "overweight" category had less risk of dying than people of normal weight.

Obese people have a greater mortality risk overall and have an increased risk of having diabetes or other conditions, but people at the lowest obesity level with a BMI of 30 to 34.9 were not more likely to die than people classified as having a normal weight. This study is not a free pass to be overweight, but people must consider all factors in determining if they are indeed at their healthiest weight.

BMI-categorized "overweight" people need not panic unless they have other indicators of poor health. Depending on where fat is in the body, it might be protective or even nutritional, particularly for older people or those who suffer from an illness.

According to Sander L. Gilman, Ph.D., a professor at Emory University in Atlanta, "The problem today seems to be that we have demonized fat…we have lowered the boundary for *overweight* to include people considered *normal* a generation ago." I mention this before you do these calculations so you have a full perspective on health and size. Just a hundred years ago, a 5'7" woman at 171 pounds was selected by the medical examiner as a woman of perfect health. Her BMI was 27—yet today's body mass index would consider her to be overweight.

If you are healthy according to your doctor but fall in the overweight BMI category, you may be actually at the perfect weight for *you*. I know a woman who is 5'6" and weighs 160 pounds, placing her in the overweight category, yet she is extremely fit and healthy. For me, at 5'7", I felt healthiest at 128 pounds. But my current over-40 weight is 138 pounds, and I can easily maintain this weight by eating like a woman. I feel great and my loved ones say I look great! On the other hand, when I went through menopause and I gained 25 pounds, my health was comprised—I experienced high blood pressure and high C-Reactive Protein (a protein found in the blood, and levels rise in response to inflammation), increasing my risk of cardiovascular disease.

Weight is highly individualized. Each of us is unique.

However, using the BMI chart can give you a healthy weight estimate based on height and weight, so go back to the BMI chart and look at the overall weights for your height in the "normal" category.

EXAMPLE: A 5'6" woman would have a normal weight range within 118 and 148 pounds.

EXAMPLE: A 5'7" woman would have a normal weight range between 121 to 153 pounds.

What Is Your Waist-to-Hip Ratio?

Using the BMI chart gives you a healthy weight estimate based on height and weight. The waist-to-hip ratio calculation will tell you if you are carrying fat in the wrong places.

To determine whether you have a healthy waist-to-hip ratio, use a fabric measuring tape and measure the circumference of your hips at the widest part of your buttocks. Then measure your waist at the smallest circumference of your natural waist, usually just above the belly button.

To determine the ratio, divide your waist measurement by your hip measurement:

_____ (waist) ÷ _____ (hip) = _____ waist-to-hip ratio

WAIST-TO-HIP RATIO CHART	
Measurement	Health Risk
0.80 or below	Low
0.81-0.85	Moderate
0.85+	High

What Are Your Body Fat Percentage and Lean Body Mass?

Next, we will calculate how many pounds of body fat and how many pounds of lean body mass (muscles, organs, bones) you are carrying, as well as your body fat percentage.

The best time to use this formula is in the morning. Your body weight and waist measurements are the most accurate just after you wake up from 7 to 8 hours of sleep.

To calculate lean body mass, body fat weight and body fat percentage, we must first collect some numbers.

1. Total body weight

_____ × 0.732 = _____ + 8.987 = _____

2. Wrist measurement at the fullest point

_____ ÷ 3.140 = _____

3. Waist measurement at your belly button

_____ × 0.157 = _____

4. Hip measurement at the fullest point

_____ × 0.249 = _____

5. Forearm measurement at the fullest point

_____ × 0.434 = _____

Once you calculate 1 through 5, use these numbers for the next three formulas.

Lean Body Mass Formula Using Calculation Numbers 1–5

1 _____ + 2 _____ − 3 _____ − 4 _____ + 5 _____

= _____ your lean body mass in pounds

Body Fat Weight Formula Using Calculation Numbers 1–5

Total body weight _____ − lean body mass (pounds) _____

= _____ your body fat weight in pounds

Body Fat Percentage

Body fat weight _____ × 100 = _____

÷ your total body weight _____

= _____ your body fat percentage

> Good news!
> EatLikeAWoman.com
> has health calculators to
> make your life easier.

Your Frame Size Relative to Weight

This chart is very helpful because it incorporates your frame size. Here's how to determine your frame size. Place your thumb and index finger around your wrist. If your finger overlaps the thumb, you have a small frame. If they touch, your frame is a medium frame. If they do not touch, you have a large frame.

WOMEN			
Height	**Frame Size**		
Feet/Inches	Small	Med	Large
4'10"	102–111	109–121	118–131
4'11"	103–113	111–123	120–134
5'0"	104–115	113–126	122–137
5'1"	106–118	115–129	125–140
5'2"	108–121	118–132	128–143
5'3"	111–124	121–135	131–147
5'4"	114–127	124–138	134–151
5'5"	117–130	127–141	137–155
5'6"	120–133	130–144	140–159
5'7"	123–136	133–147	143–163

Height	Frame Size		
Feet/Inches	Small	Med	Large
5′8″	126–139	136–150	146–167
5′9″	129–142	139–153	149–170
5′10″	132–145	142–156	152–173
5′11″	135–148	145–159	155–176
6′0″	138–151	148–162	158–179

Having your body fat calculated underwater by a professional will give the most accurate measurement. I have never done this, and most of us will not have this opportunity, but using the BMI chart, waist-to-hip ratio, and body fat and lean muscle mass calculations then noting your weight range from the frame size chart above can give you a healthy weight range to be used for your *Eat Like a Woman* plan.

Are Your Meds Making You Fat?

For years I struggled with allergies, and Benadryl was my favorite drug of choice. I used it to manage hives, to avoid a reaction when around cats and to get some sleep when stressed because it always knocked me out. As the years passed, I took it almost every day.

Years later, those 24-hour over-the-counter, nondrowsy antihistamines became readily available, and I lived on those drugs. Every year, a few new extra pounds started showing up on the scale. I assumed it was the natural part of aging, despite my level of physical activity. Then, once I hit menopause, my blood pressure skyrocketed, and my health-care provider put me on hypertension drugs. My health-care provider confirmed the antihistamines and hypertension drugs were contributing to weight gain, but unhealthy lifestyle choices were also part of the problem.

There is a pill for almost every problem, but many drugs, including diabetes medicines, may be contributing to weight gain. There are drugs listed by the World Health Organization used in the treatment of chronic health problems that are associated with weight gain as a side effect and are considered "obesogenic."

The following list describes some of these drugs and how they can lead to weight gain:

DRUGS THAT CAN MAKE YOU GAIN WEIGHT

DRUG	USED FOR
Antidepressants: Some antidepressants may trigger food cravings. The selected serotonin reuptake inhibitor (SSRI) Paxil is the most likely to cause weight gain, while another SSRI, Zoloft, is the least likely. Bupropion (Wellbutrin) is a dopamine agonist and does not increase weight.	Depression
Benadryl, Allegra, Zyrtec: One study found that those taking Allegra and Zyrtec were 55% more likely to be overweight than those not taking the drugs. Histamine, a chemical found in some of the body's cells that causes many of the symptoms of allergies, signals our bodies to regulate our appetites so that we don't overeat. According to the study, we inadvertently turn this process off when taking antihistamines to reduce allergy symptoms, thus allowing us to overeat and gain weight.	Allergy
Beta-blockers: Older beta-blockers caused weight gain in the first few months of use by slowing calorie burning and causing fatigue. New beta-blockers, ACE (angiotensin-converting-enzyme) inhibitors and calcium channel blockers are less likely to cause weight gain.	Hypertension
Corticosteroids: These treatments can increase appetite, slow down metabolism and lead to extra deposits of fat on the body, especially around the abdomen. Some gain anywhere from 20 to 40 pounds when using them.	Inflammatory disease

DRUG	USED FOR
Cyproheptadine: This may increase appetite, resulting in weight gain. There may also be a small sedative effect that could contribute to a decrease in activity, resulting in weight gain.	Allergy, hay fever
Insulin: This medication can increase hunger; some gain up to 11 pounds during the first three years of use. In addition, sulphonylureas lowers blood sugar and may increase appetite; thiazolinidiones can cause fluid retention in the body and weight gain.	Diabetes
Lithium: Weight gain during the first year of treatment occurred in 47% of the women but only 18% of the men. Lithium causes a slow but steady weight gain. It can cause hypothyroidism, and hypothyroidism can cause weight gain. Also, lithium causes thirst (by acting in your system rather like the sodium in table salt). If you respond to that thirst with sugared drinks, you have added a significant source of calories to your daily intake.	Bipolar disorder
Sodium valproate: Females are more prone to gain weight when using this drug. The drug affects proteins involved in appetite and metabolism, although it's not clear why it appears to affect women more than men.	Epilepsy
Statins: These medications can cause muscle cramps, limiting activity and exercise, thus leading to weight gain because you are not burning calories.	Cholesterol
Tamoxifen: This drug can increase appetite.	Breast cancer

Most of the medications mentioned here may contribute to significant weight gain, and if you take a combination of these obesogenic drugs, additional pounds may occur.

What's not on this list? Birth control pills! Birth control pills (estradiol and progestin) are often blamed for weight gain, but this is unproven in the research literature. However, progestin-only contraceptives, such as Depo-Provera and Norplant, generally do cause weight gain.

It should be noted that being ill can cause stress, and stress can pack on the pounds, too. Chronic stress can be tied to an *increase* in appetite, causing stress-induced weight gain. This type of weight gain has the tendency to store "visceral fat" around the midsection. These fat cells that lie deep within the abdomen have been linked to an increase in both diabetes and heart disease.

Discuss your medications and any weight gain concerns with your health-care provider. For many, decreasing your calorie intake by just 100 to 200 calories per day combined with daily exercise can counteract weight gain from some of these drugs. By eating just 100 extra calories per day—that's like two saltine crackers—for over a month, you have consumed 3,000 extra calories. That is equal to one pound of fat. Before making any changes to your medications, speak with your doctor.

Assuming that medications are not contributing to weight gain, a recent study published in the *Journal of Nutritional Biochemistry* revealed that exercise was more effective in reducing fat, while dieting is more effective in reducing weight in healthy women. The *Eat Like a Woman* program harnesses this science to encourage overall health.

Accepting Our Differences and Our Bodies

Having a positive body image can fuel healthy choices. Having healthy weight expectations for your body size, frame and genetics can boost self-esteem, allowing you the freedom to focus on your dreams, not your weight.

The *Eat Like a Woman* philosophy embraces the fact that women biologically and genetically have more fat for reproduction and survival than men. We must manage our food intake and activity to achieve overall health for each life stage.

2

The *Eat Like a Woman* 3-Step, 3-Week Plan

Chapter 7

Step 1

How to Eat Like a Woman

Are you eating like a woman or like a man?

YES	NO	DO YOU PREFER?
		Eggs more than ham
		Cinnamon more than horseradish
		Frozen carrots more than frozen pizza
		Grilled chicken more than sirloin steak
		Almonds more than peanuts
		Berries and cream more than jalapeño peppers
		Smooth peanut butter more than crunchy peanut butter
		Tomatoes more than asparagus
		Buying fresh ground beef more than frozen
		Brussels sprouts more than green beans
		Eggs scrambled more than sunny-side up

If you answered yes to all or most of the above, you eat like a woman. Recent research conducted by the Infectious Disease Society of America surveyed 14,878 persons and revealed there are indeed sex-based differences in food consumption.

In this survey, women had a greater likelihood of eating fruits and vegetables. Men were more likely to eat meat. Women chose sweeter flavors over spicier and tended to eat less risky foods such as undercooked eggs. Considering that in the latter half of our monthly cycle, the luteal phase, women respond more strongly to food smells and desire high-fat foods, it is no surprise that we love our sweet treats.

Many believe our gendered diet can be explained by evolution. Some say it's cultural. Either way, the fact is women and men tend to gravitate toward different foods. Personally, when I wait too long to eat and my blood sugar crashes, I'll grab anything in the carbohydrate department, but my husband reaches for protein. One thing is for sure: our DNA is the same as that of our cave(wo)man ancestors.

Women are programmed to eat based on scarcity. When food was in front of you, you ate because you didn't know when the next meal would be popping up from the earth. When we walk into our modern kitchens stocked with lots of food, we hit the food jackpot and eat! In other words, our supply chain in the 21st century is abundant, but the programming to eat when food is available contributes to overconsumption and subsequent weight gain.

With our modern-day abundance of food and our automated society, it is no surprise that obesity is such an epidemic. We have engineered physical activity out of our lives. Throw in sugar, high-fructose corn syrup (HFCS), refined grains, processed foods, grain-fed animals, and added fats, this unhealthy consumption has yielded diseases that never existed in the days of our ancestors.

How do we survive in such a hostile food environment today and still honor our bodies as women? Awareness is the first step. Action is the next step.

There are many confusing messages about what to eat or not eat surrounding us. For many, these bombarding messages, combined with images of the perfect body, contribute to yo-yo dieting, fueling the diet industry's success and our loss of self-esteem. How can one message or one plan apply to everyone? We are all different, yet our basic needs as women are the same.

Research shows that a woman's brain doesn't signal her to stop eating when she is full as well as a man's brain, and this may contribute to overeating and subsequent obesity.

The word *diet* comes from the Greek root *diatia* and the Latin *diaeta*, which mean "to live one's life"! *Eat Like a Woman* is a lifestyle that celebrates life.

All humans need protein, carbohydrates, fats and water to survive. However, in this section of *Eat Like a Woman*, we will explore food choices that support our health as women. From hormones to neurotransmitters to our digestive system and fat cells, I have taken the science of sex-based differences and applied them to a woman's health through each life stage.

How the sexes differ in the way that they absorb and process nutrients is only beginning to be fully studied, so the information presented here is based on the science that is available to date. So let's feed our differences so we look and feel great!

Today we know that heart disease symptoms are very different between women and men. Bone health also differs, and dosing of some medications is different for men and women. How the sexes absorb and process nutrients is only beginning to be fully studied.

Protein Power

Your hormones and neurotransmitters love protein! Protein is essential for the growth and repair of body tissues, can be used to provide energy during starvation and acts as bodybuilding materials. Your skin, muscles, hair and nails are made up of proteins.

The benefits of protein are many:

1. Protein is digested more slowly from the stomach to the intestine. This makes you feel full longer, stabilizing the effect of food on blood sugar. Unstable blood sugar levels affect your mood and hormones.

2. Consuming protein low in saturated fat can improve your blood triglycerides and high-density lipoprotein. Lower cholesterol and triglycerides can reduce your risk of heart attack or stroke.

3. Protein is indispensable for the growth and maintenance of the cells in our body.

4. Proteins in the form of enzymes, antibodies and hormones can promote a strong, healthy metabolic process, which could boost your nervous and immune systems.

Today we know that women absorb medications differently than men, but there is little science available on nutrient absorption. A recent study published in *Nutrition, Metabolism and Cardiovascular Diseases* revealed interesting information regarding the absorption of the omega-3 fatty acids EPA and DHA.

EPA and DHA are converted into hormone-like substances called prostaglandins, which play a role in regulating cell activity and promoting healthy cardiovascular function. EPA benefits cardiovascular health due to its anti-coagulation ability (blood thinning). DHA has little effect on cellular inflammation, but is an important nutrient for pregnant women, and helps healthy fetal brain development. It is critical during the first 6 months of life for proper nervous system as well as visual development.

Males may benefit more from EPA supplementation while females may gain more from DHA, suggesting a possible need for a change in the way omega-3s are delivered in dietary supplements. New omega-3 fatty acid research is in the pipeline exploring sex differences in absorption. In the meantime, follow your health-care provider's recommendation and stay tuned for updates on omega-3 supplementation for each sex.

5. Our body development, healing of wounds, replacement of dead cells, hair and nail growth, and the replenishment of lost blood is dependent on protein.

Consuming high-protein, high-fiber snack bars may reduce your overall food intake and improve your short-term glucose and insulin profile. Not consuming enough protein can lead to weakening of the muscles, heart and respiratory system; growth loss; decreased immunity; and even death.

Complete vs. Incomplete Proteins

All the neurotransmitters, with the exception of acetylcholine, are made from amino acids with the help of minerals, vitamins and other nutrients. Your body breaks down dietary protein into amino acids.

There are two groups of proteins: complete proteins and incomplete proteins. Proteins consumed from animal sources (meat, fish, poultry, milk, cheese and eggs) are **complete proteins**. They contain the necessary essential amino acids for human use. The only exception is soy (a plant source); it is also considered a complete protein. Amino acids are the chemical building blocks from which new proteins are made, so consuming complete proteins is important.

Grains, legumes, seeds, nuts and a variety of other foods are **incomplete proteins** because they provide only some of the essential amino acids. Fortunately for our vegan and vegetarian sisters, combining different incomplete proteins makes it possible to obtain all necessary amino acids. For example, combining rice and beans makes a complete protein.

Some amino acids come from food, some are made in the body and some are converted from the other amino acids. If we don't have a sufficient supply of amino acids, we may not have the components that are essential for the production of neurotransmitters in the brain and in the gut.

There are many things that can deplete neurotransmitter levels:

- Excess caffeine
- Too much nicotine
- Mineral depletion
- Vitamin depletion
- Excess alcohol

A busy lifestyle can be loaded with daily stressors. Some of us enjoy a few glasses of wine or a cigarette to relax. Others grab sweet treats or comforting junk food. All these habits help us survive the stress of the modern world but can compromise the health of our neurotransmitters. Once you begin to eat like a woman, you can balance your food intake to help the neurotransmitter system so you feel better while functioning in this hectic world.

There are certain foods that contain starting materials for neurotransmitters called precursors. If a diet is deficient in precursors, the brain will not be able to produce some neurotransmitters. Neurological and mental disorders may occur when the balance of neurotransmitters is upset. More on this later.

Protein and the Thermic Effect

Protein has a wonderful hidden benefit called the thermic effect. Your body uses 60 to 75 percent of its energy for basic functions (breathing, heartbeat). Physical activity also uses energy, and you use energy during the digestion process called the thermic effect of food. Some of the foods you eat speed up your metabolism.

Dietary fat is easy to process and has little thermic effect, but protein is harder to process so it has a larger thermic effect. It takes extra energy, up to 30 percent more, to break down protein into amino acids and glucose, and to synthesize new proteins in your body.

Our bodies are designed to bear children, but in our modern world, we now have a choice about when, if and how many children we want. We are no longer pregnant during most of our reproductive years, even though our bodies are still programmed for this. Since our bodies are built to grab every morsel of carbs and fats, why not utilize protein to balance our new environment?

Upping your protein intake can often kick-start your weight-loss program, but it is not good for the long haul. Many believe in high-protein diets that restrict carb intake for life, but they may be at risk for nutritional deficiencies or insufficient fiber.

> Spicy foods and caffeine can stimulate the thermic effect of food. Studies claim that the active ingredient in chili (capsaicin) can increase diet-induced thermogenesis by over 50 percent, which over time may cumulate to help weight loss and prevent weight gain.

In addition, eating too much red meat and full-fat dairy products may increase the risk of heart disease or worsen kidney function in people with kidney disease because the body may have trouble eliminating all the waste products of protein metabolism.

If you decide to jump-start weight loss by incorporating the thermic effect of protein, choose your protein wisely: fish, skinless chicken, lean beef, pork and low-fat dairy products are good choices.

Talk to your health-care provider before starting a high-protein weight-loss strategy, especially if you have kidney or liver disease, diabetes, or other chronic health conditions.

See Appendix A for a list of healthy proteins.

Carbohydrates

Carbohydrates are your brain's primary fuel source and your body's chief source of energy. You don't need carbohydrates to survive, but without them you could feel crabby and fatigued. Carbs provide fuel, but your body can produce energy from proteins and fat alone.

Types of Carbohydrates

There are basically two types of carbohydrates.

Sugars are simple carbohydrates that provide instant energy. Simple carbohydrates have small molecules and are digested quickly. Many products processed and prepared with refined sugar are simple carbs (white sugar, pastas made with white flour, bread made with white flour, fruit juice, cakes, chocolate, soda, biscuits). These are not "friendly" carbs for gals struggling to obtain a healthy weight or in a life stage with fluctuating hormones. But *natural* simple carbohydrates such as apples, cherries, lemons, melons, oranges, peaches and strawberries are great to consume if you are trying to regain control over your weight. Other simple carbs are dairy products. Low-fat dairy products are healthy choices for your food plan.

Starches are complex carbohydrates. Whole-grain breads, oatmeal, muesli, brown rice, whole-wheat pasta, potatoes, starchy vegetables (corn, peas), and legumes (beans, lentils) are complex carbohydrates. Complex carbs take the body longer to digest because they have larger molecules. Because this process takes longer, your energy lasts longer. Complex carbs often provide sources of fiber—some wonderful sources for this are fruits (apples, pears, strawberries), vegetables (carrots, spinach, zucchini), whole grains, whole-grain bread, whole-grain pastas and cereals. These are "friendly" carbs if consumed in moderation.

Understanding the difference between "good" and "bad" carbs can be an important step to maintaining a healthy weight and overall health through the life stages.

Carbohydrates and Blood Sugar

After consuming carbohydrates, your body turns them into glucose—blood sugar. As women, maintaining steady blood sugar levels is important to our hormone and neurotransmitter health, and your blood sugar level can affect your mood and overall health.

The glycemic index (GI) was created in the 1980s. The GI classifies carbs based on how quickly they are digested and how high they boost blood sugar compared to pure glucose. Using the GI is a wonderful tool supported by science to manage your metabolism, weight and hormones! What's great about using the GI is you are not eliminating foods but only swapping them.

If you struggle with type 1 or type 2 diabetes, hypoglycemia, or being overweight or obese, or if you have high levels of triglycerides, belly fat or polycystic ovarian syndrome (PCOS), incorporating the GI into your food planning will benefit your health. Eating low-glycemic foods can assist in weight management through each life stage and control type 2 diabetes.

The glycemic load is a way to classify foods that takes into account both the amount and the quality of the carbohydrates that they contain. Foods that are high in rapidly digested carbohydrates—a can of sugary soda, a handful of jelly beans, a plateful of pasta—have a high glycemic load and can cause dramatic peaks in your blood sugar. Eating a diet rich in high-glycemic foods may, over time, lead to type 2 diabetes, heart disease and other conditions.

However, eating low-glycemic foods like high-fiber breakfast cereals (made of wheat bran, oats and/or barley), lentils, baked beans, veggies and fruit causes a more gentle change in blood sugar.

Eating low-glycemic carbs has many benefits:

+ Blood sugar levels in your body are sustained for longer periods of time.

+ Your hunger urges are controlled because the blood sugar levels are slowly being released into your bloodstream.

+ You are able to exercise for longer periods of time.

+ Your risk of getting type 2 diabetes and heart disease are reduced.

+ Your cholesterol levels will be under control.

+ Most low-glycemic foods are lower in calories and fat.

> According to the Academy of Nutrition and Dietetics, in healthy women, small amounts of cinnamon result in lower blood glucose levels after a meal. It is not a magic potion to lose weight, but it can be a wonderful way to help balance blood sugar levels. Better yet, replace refined sugar with cinnamon—a yummy, healthy choice!

+ Many low-glycemic foods are loaded with fiber and nutrients.
+ These foods can be a useful meal-planning tool for weight loss during menopause.

Consumption of lean proteins combined with low- to medium-glycemic carbs has been found to assist weight loss for women going through menopause. I can personally confirm this finding, as its inclusion in *The Menopause Makeover* formula has helped women worldwide lose weight. Now the science confirms it!

If you consume high-glycemic carbs, combine that food with a low-glycemic food. For example, if you eat corn flakes for breakfast (high GI), add some strawberries (low GI) to make it a medium-glycemic value.

The following is a list of possible low-glycemic substitutes (in the "Hello" column) that can be used to replace their high-glycemic counterparts (in the "Bye Bye" column):

CARBOHYDRATE SWAPS

BYE BYE	HELLO
White bread	100% whole-wheat bread
White rice	Brown rice
White potatoes	Yams
White pasta	Whole-wheat pasta
Sugary cereals	Oatmeal

See the Healthy Carbohydrates Using the Glycemic Index section in Appendix A for further guidance.

Fat

Your body needs a certain amount of fat to function, and in moderate amounts, fat is not bad for you, as discussed in Chapter 6. It transports oxygen to every cell in your body, it is a component for building cells and body tissue, and absorbing some vitamins and other nutrients, and it is also the basis for your hormones, brain, and nervous system. The good fats can protect you from cancer.

Fats are classified as animal fats (butter, milk, ghee, fish, meat) or vegetable fats (sunflower oil, sesame oil). Sources of good fats come from fish, egg yolks, nuts, seeds, olives and unrefined oils (extra-virgin oils).

There are three naturally occurring types of fats: polyunsaturated, monounsaturated and saturated. And there is one man-made fat: trans fat.

The Good Fats

There are essentially two good kinds of fats: polyunsaturated and monounsaturated (see Appendix A for a list of good fats).

Polyunsaturated fats include the omega-3 fats found in fish oil. Polyunsaturated fish oils can protect the heart by lowering triglyceride levels and preventing blood clots. Natural sources of omega-3 fats can be found in salmon, sardines, herring and rainbow trout.

Fish and fish oils have also been shown to be a great mood stabilizer, as well as ease depression, lower cholesterol, reduce inflammation, eliminate joint pain, improve complexion and promote weight loss.

If you are not a fish lover, you can also find omega-3 fats in flaxseed, soybeans, chia seeds, walnuts, almonds, pistachios, dark leafy greens, and canola and soy oils.

Omega-6 is another good fat. Your body cannot produce omega-6; it must be obtained from foods. It can be found in olive oil, chicken, eggs, avocado, chia seeds, pumpkin seeds, acai berries, soybean oil, corn oil, sunflower oil and cottonseed oil. Omega-6 fats are great for your skin and hair.

Monounsaturated fats are the healthiest fat choice, as they can help you reduce your blood cholesterol when substituted for saturated fats. Olive oil, canola oil, peanut oil, macadamia oils, almonds, peanuts, pecans, cashews and avocados contain monounsaturated fats. Vegetable oil fats remain liquid at room temperature and are one of the healthiest oils to add to your food plan.

Monounsaturated fats can lower your bad cholesterol (LDL) levels and increase your good cholesterol (HDL) levels. Stock your house with extra-virgin olive oil, almonds, grass-fed meats, nuts, sesame oil and avocados. If cooking at high temperatures, use canola oil, and when baking, use canola oil instead of shortening, margarine or other oils.

> Dietary cholesterol is produced naturally by the body and is also found in foods that are derived from animals. It tends to raise blood cholesterol in individuals who don't eat balanced meals.

> The consumption of virgin olive oil as part of a Mediterranean diet may protect against bone loss in the elderly. It is okay to cook with olive oil, but do not use it for deep-frying.

The Bad Fats

Just as there are good fats, there are bad fats: saturated and trans fats.

Saturated fat is found in red meat and other animal products such as dairy products, cheese, sour cream, ice cream, butter and lard, as well as tropical oils such as coconut oil, coconut milk, cocoa butter and palm oils. They remain solid at room temperature. Saturated fats raise LDL (bad) cholesterol levels, which can lead to hardening of the arteries and contribute to blood clots; in turn, blood vessels can become clogged, which can result in a stroke or heart attack. The saturated fatty acids myristic acid and palmitic acid are found in cream, butter, and some meats and are associated with a higher risk of heart disease.

However, despite their bad reputation, saturated fats are under the microscope again, because they are not all the same, and some sources are shown to have many health benefits. Limited amounts of whole-food saturated fat sources, such as eggs, butter and grass-fed meat, may not be as bad as we once thought, especially when intake is balanced with plenty of anti-inflammatory omega-3s and phytonutrients from vegetables and fruits.

Similarly, coconut oil has a saturated fat called lauric acid, which may actually reduce high cholesterol by promoting its conversion to pregnenolone, a molecule that is a precursor to many of the hormones our bodies need. Some studies report that coconut oil eaters were shown to have a higher level of "good" HDL, which helps clear cholesterol deposits from arteries. There is emerging research that claims it is also good for the immunity and digestion, and it may aid with weight loss.

The saturated fats present in coconut oil have antimicrobial properties and can help fight some bacteria, parasites and fungi that may lead to indigestion. Coconut oil can also help absorption of other nutrients. There are also some claims that coconut oil is useful for managing Alzheimer's disease and helps in the brain function.

Not all coconut oil is created equal, though. It's important to purchase coconut oil that is 100 percent organic and extra virgin. While many claim the coconut can be a superfood, the jury is still out on coconut oil. There is no solid evidence that coconut oil can decrease your heart disease risk, boost your immune system or help you lose weight. Therefore, don't substitute it for other beneficial oils, such as olive oil.

Trans fat is a hydrogenated fat that is man-made, created by adding hydrogen to a polyunsaturated fat, turning liquid oils into more solid fats such as margarine. Trans fats can be found in baked goods, fried foods, donuts, French fries, crackers and snacks. Trans fats raise your LDL (bad) cholesterol levels and lower HDL (good) cholesterol levels. The American Heart Association recommends an intake of less than 1 percent of total calories via trans fats per day. Scientific evidence shows that the consumption of saturated fats and trans fats increases the risk of coronary heart disease.

Fabulous Fiber

Fiber is found in all fruits, grains, vegetables and legumes. Fiber is usually found in the outer layer of the plant and is considered to be a carbohydrate. Fiber cannot be digested, so when you eat fiber, it passes through your body virtually unchanged.

Fiber is broken down into two categories: insoluble and soluble. Insoluble fiber, found in wheat bran and many veggies such as celery, cannot be dissolved in water and passes through the digestive system, absorbing water and adding bulk to stool. Soluble fiber, found in oatmeal, barley, kidney beans, and some fruits and veggies, can dissolve in water, forming a gel in the intestines.

Fiber has many benefits. Eating fiber:

- Keeps your bowels regular and stools soft.
- Moves fat through your digestive system quicker, an added benefit for battling menopause's mid-section belly fat.
- Can help you lose weight.
- Leaves you feeling full longer.
- Keeps your blood sugar on an even keel.
- Can transport bad cholesterol out of your body, which is good for heart health.
- Can reduce the risk of certain diseases (heart disease, diabetes).

You should consume 21 to 25 grams of fiber per day (see Appendix A for a list of healthy fiber choices.) Fiber is a wonderful part of your diet. Keep that plumbing clean!

Eating to Increase Your Neurotransmitter Health

As previously discussed in Chapter 3, your diet has an important effect on your neurotransmitters and that can affect how you feel. Let's see how.

Serotonin

Have you been feeling cranky and blah? Many of us grab sweets or high-glycemic carbohydrates to feel better, but this can actually lead to decreased sensitivity to the neurotransmitter serotonin, leading to an even worse mood and increasing your odds of gaining weight. Here's how you can increase your serotonin precursors so you feel good, sleep well and enjoy a healthy self-esteem.

1. **Consume foods high in tryptophan.** The starting point for stabilizing serotonin levels is to eat foods that have plenty of the amino acid tryptophan, which the body converts to serotonin. Try to include at least one tryptophan-rich food at every meal, choosing organic foods whenever possible.

The following foods have high amounts of tryptophan:

- Turkey
- Fish: tuna, salmon, shrimp
- Chicken
- Lean pork
- Veal
- Wild game meats
- Lamb
- Bananas
- Milk
- Yogurt
- Eggs
- Cottage cheese
- Swiss and cheddar cheese
- Nuts: peanuts, hazelnuts, walnuts, almonds
- Beans: lentils, peanuts, garbanzo beans
- Avocados
- Wheat germ

> Here is a warning for some migraine sufferers: tryptophans can be headache triggers. Also, if you are taking monoamine oxidase inhibitors, you should avoid foods high in tryptophans.

Serotonin is synthesized from tryptophan in the presence of adequate vitamins: thiamin-B_1 (found in asparagus, tuna, flaxseeds, green peas and Brussels sprouts), niacin-B_3 (found in chicken, tuna, turkey, halibut and salmon), B_6 (found in bell peppers, summer squash, turnip greens, shiitake mushrooms, spinach, tuna and beef), and folic acid (found in romaine lettuce, spinach, asparagus, mustard greens, parsley, broccoli, cauliflower, beets and lentils).

2. **Consume carbohydrates.** Good news! Your carb cravings do have a good purpose. A carbohydrate snack raises insulin levels, which ushers the precursor to serotonin, the amino acid tryptophan, into the brain.

The healthiest carbohydrates to eat are whole grains; low- to medium-glycemic index carbohydrates, such as barley, oats and buckwheat; and carbohydrate-rich vegetables, such as yams, sweet potatoes and squashes.

> Men are 52 percent more effective in absorbing tryptophan than women, perhaps explaining the fact that many of us women eat more sweets and junk food to feel better.

3. **Avoid the stimulant cycle.** Many of us get trapped in the stimulant cycle and overconsume caffeine, sugar and alcohol. These substances temporarily give you a lift, but continually consuming them for this purpose can lead to a destructive habit. If you like caffeine, try to limit this pick-me-up to one or two cups a day at the most. The same for alcohol, though one serving of red wine has been shown to have some health benefits.

In the early stages of serotonin deficiency, proper diet and exercise can assist with the serotonin imbalance within just a couple of months.

Dopamine, Norepinephrine and Epinephrine

Dopamine is derived from the amino acids phenylalanine and tyrosine, and dopamine is the precursor to norepinephrine and epinephrine. Here's how to promote dopamine, norepinephrine and epinephrine production for alertness and energy:

1. **Eat foods rich in phenylalanine.** Some sources are:

- Beef
- Poultry: turkey, chicken
- Pork
- Fish: salmon, cod, trout
- Milk
- Yogurt
- Eggs
- Cheese
- Soy products (including soy protein isolate, soybean flour and tofu)
- Dry whole lentils
- Nuts: almonds, peanuts
- Seeds: sesame, pumpkin
- Wheat germ

2. **Eat foods full of tyrosine.** Some sources are:

- Beef
- Poultry: turkey, chicken
- Pork
- Eggs
- Cheese: Parmesan, Gouda, mozzarella, Swiss, ricotta
- Fish: cod
- Oysters
- Seeds: sesame, pumpkin
- Nuts: almonds
- Soybeans and tofu
- Milk
- Bananas
- Avocados
- Lima beans

3. **Include Vitamin B$_6$.** Wheat germ, tuna, almond butter, poultry, legumes, soy and noncitrus fruits such as watermelon and bananas are all excellent sources of vitamin B$_6$.

4. **Find folic acid.** Your mother was right in encouraging you to eat spinach, broccoli and legumes, as these foods are rich in folic acid.

5. **Get enough copper.** Consuming shellfish, whole grains, prunes, beans, nuts and seeds will see to your copper needs.

6. **Drink green tea.** A substance in green tea, theanine, has been shown to trigger the release of dopamine.

Gamma Aminobutyric Acid

Gamma Aminobutyric Acid (GABA) is critical to help manage stress, maintain mental focus and regulate the body's internal rhythm. The amino acid glutamine is derived from glutamate and is necessary for the production of GABA. If you have a GABA deficiency that is mild to moderate, you should be able to balance it with diet, exercise and lifestyle modifications. Here's how to make sure your diet is contributing to your GABA health:

1. **Seek foods high in glutamate.** Some good sources are:

⬧ Almonds	⬧ Brown rice	⬧ Oranges, citrus fruits
⬧ Tree nuts	⬧ Halibut	⬧ Rice bran
⬧ Bananas	⬧ Lentils	⬧ Spinach
⬧ Beef liver	⬧ Oats	⬧ Walnuts
⬧ Broccoli	⬧ Whole grains	

2. **Eat healthy complex carbohydrates.** These will increase glutamate, which forms glutamine.

3. **Drink green tea.** A substance in green tea called theanine can help improve mood and create a sense of relaxation. Theanine induces the release of GABA, according to a Chinese study conducted in 2012.

Acetylcholine

Unlike the other neurotransmitters, acetylcholine is not made from amino acids. Its primary building block is choline, which belongs to the B family of vitamins. Here's how to increase acetylcholine levels for better memory and concentration:

1. **Eat foods high in choline.** Egg yolks, wheat germ, soybeans, organ meats (liver, brain, heart, tongue and tripe), and whole-wheat products are high in choline. In addition, eggs contain cholesterol essential for the machinery that triggers the release of this neurotransmitter, increasing neurotransmitter function by five times.

2. **Use the herb rosemary.** Rosemary contains several compounds that prevent the breakdown of acetylcholine.

3. **Avoid toxins.** Aluminum toxicity, Polycholorinated biphenyl (PCBs), chemical fertilizers, pesticides and electromagnetic fields are all detrimental to acetylcholine.

Extra Brain Health Tips

Here are some additional tips for the feeding and care of your neurotransmitters.

1. **Control your caffeine intake.** Studies support the safety of a cup or two of coffee a day, and it may lower the incidence of depression. However, more than that can begin to have counter-productive effects in some people. Keep in mind that this tip is not permission to load up on coffee drinks that are loaded with sugar, cream and syrup.

2. **Moderate your alcohol intake.** One drink a day may be linked with better overall health as women age, according to a number of studies. The benefits of red wine are numerous:

+ It may lower your cholesterol.
+ It may protect your heart.
+ Its natural compound, resveratrol, may actually help regulate blood sugar.
+ Polyphenol, an extract from the red grapes used to make red wine, can boost brainpower by keeping your memory sharp.
+ It contains antioxidants, which, according to the National Health Institutes, are believed to fight infection and protect cells.
+ It helps you maintain a healthy weight. The *Journal of Biological Chemistry* published research findings suggesting that piceatannol (a compound that our body converts from resveratrol) can actually prevent the growth of fat cells.

The association between drinking and good health was even more pronounced in women who spread out their drinking—for example, one drink five nights a week, rather than several drinks a few times during the week. However, women who consume two to five drinks daily have 1.5 times the risk of developing breast cancer than non-drinkers, and even women who consume one drink daily have "a very small" increase in risk. Therefore, be sure to consume alcohol in moderation. Moderate alcohol consumption is defined as having up to one drink per day for women—here is what "one drink" translates into:

* 12 ounces of beer (approx. 150–200 calories)
* 8 ounces of malt liquor (100–200 calories)
* 5 ounces of wine (150–200 calories)
* 1.5 ounces or a "shot" of 80-proof distilled spirits or liquor (e.g., gin, rum, vodka or whiskey; 100–150 calories)

Drinking alcohol during a meal is associated with making poor food choices or skipping meals altogether. (I don't know about you, but once I have a martini, that breadbasket starts calling my name. Fortunately, red wine does not have this effect on me.) Remember, alcohol has calories. Adults get almost as many empty calories from booze as from soft drinks. That said, if you enjoy a cocktail during mealtime, make sure you are surrounded by good food choices.

3. **Drink water.** The brain is composed of 70 to 90 percent water. Water is needed for the brain's production of neurotransmitters.

4. **Eat small meals.** Throughout the day, eat several small meals so that you manage hunger, blood sugar and emotional health. If you are hungry or cranky from low blood sugar, making healthy lifestyle decisions that can affect your neurotransmitter health is more challenging.

5. **Eat healthy fats.** Focus on eating healthy fats, such as those found in salmon, whitefish, flounder, trout, fish oil supplements, walnuts, flaxseeds, olive oil and avocados to improve the sensitivity and function of neurotransmitter receptors that are responsible for problem solving, attention and mental clarity.

6. **Eat more raw foods.** Eating raw foods will help your neurotransmitters because overcooking foods can destroy essential amino acids such as tryptophan and increase the amounts of free glutamate in foods.

7. **Eat blueberries.** They help neurons in your brain communicate with one another more effectively; theoretically, this could slow memory loss.

8. **Eat iron-rich food.** Iron helps the body carry oxygen to the brain. Try to consume plenty of lean red meat, fortified breakfast cereals, dark leafy veggies, beans and lentils. Younger women tend to be more at risk of low iron due to menstrual cycles and blood loss.

Eating to Support Hormonal Health

We learned about the endocrine system and the important role of various glands and hormones in Chapter 2. Now let's talk about how to eat to keep those glands and hormones healthy and balanced.

You'll remember that the **pineal gland** is responsible for melatonin, which helps regulate sleep and wake cycles. If you have sleep issues, enjoy foods rich in tryptophan: chicken, turkey, tuna, soybeans, salmon, lamb, pork, halibut, shrimp, cod, eggs, dairy products, oatmeal, milk, russet potatoes, bananas, nuts, seeds and legumes. Combine such foods with a low- to medium-glycemic carb (low-fat string cheese, brown rice, whole-wheat bread) to encourage a restful sleep.

The **thyroid** regulates growth and development through the rate of metabolism. There's not really a specific diet that will boost your thyroid function, but healthy eating habits in general will support a healthy thyroid.

The **parathyroids** play a critical role in maintaining levels of calcium and vitamin D. Consuming the correct amount of calcium and vitamin D throughout each life stage is important.

At a recent North American Menopause Society conference, I had the privilege of meeting JoAnn E. Manson, M.D., Dr.P.H., N.C.M.P., from Brigham and Women's Hospital who is a pioneer in women's health and a leader in calcium and vitamin D studies. Regarding calcium intake, Dr. Manson says,

> *Current recommendations for calcium intake call for 1,000 mg per day for women ages 19–50 and 1,200 mg per day for women over age 50 to ensure bone health. Given recent concerns that calcium supplements may raise the risk for cardiovascular disease and kidney stones, women should aim to meet this recommendation primarily by eating a calcium-rich diet and taking calcium supplements only if needed to reach the RDA goal which is often only 500 mg per day in supplements if required.*

Calcium-containing compounds are the second most popular supplement among adults in the United States, yet most of these supplements are taken without a recommendation from a physician. As Dr. Manson points out, it is better to get your daily calcium by eating a calcium-rich diet. Food sources for calcium include dairy products; canned oily fish with bones, such as sardines or salmon; tofu; calcium-fortified juice and cereals; broccoli; collard greens; and kale.

By the age of 18, roughly 85 to 90 percent of bone mass is acquired, also known as peak bone mass, and bone formation is almost complete. In order to maximize bone health, it is critical for girls to get enough calcium and vitamin D in their diets at an early age.

In fact, the latest studies state that vitamin D, not calcium, is principally responsible for preserving bone and preventing osteoporosis among women, so ingestion of vitamin D-rich foods is critical. Foods high in vitamin D include fortified dairy products, fortified foods and fatty fish (tuna, salmon). Your skin absorbs vitamin D when exposed to sunlight of a sufficient intensity.

The **adrenals** release hormones in response to stress and produce androgens. Eating a healthy diet, avoiding sugars, moderate alcohol consumption, proper meal timing and drinking plenty of water can help maintain healthy adrenals.

The **ovaries** play an important role in development and reproduction for women. A new study of women ages 18 to 44 found that drinking coffee and other caffeinated beverages can alter levels of estrogen, but the impact varies by race. In white women, for example, coffee appears to lower estrogen, while in Asian women, it has the reverse effect, raising levels of the hormone. Drinking excessive alcohol can increase the body's conversion of testosterone into estrogen, especially in fat cells. Hormone-enhanced food products, such as soy foods (tofu, soybeans, soy veggie burgers, soy hotdogs, soy milk) that contain phytoestrogens, can also raise estrogen levels. Flaxseeds are another wonderful option loaded with phytoestrogens, as is the herb black cohosh, as well as lentils, navy, pinto and fava beans.

The **pancreas**, you will recall, secretes enzymes needed for digestion. Diets high in fatty meats, cholesterol and fried foods increase the risk of both pancreatic cancer and pancreatitis, while diets high in raw fruits and vegetables and lean proteins reduce that risk.

Not only are there sex differences in food preferences (how we absorb and taste food), but taking the latest science and applying it to our lifestyle can improve our health and how we feel at each life stage. What you eat can help you feel and look better by supporting hormonal and digestive health.

I love the new science on women and food, but it can be overwhelming and confusing. With many conflicting reports, many no longer know what food choices to make. The *Eat Like a Woman* program can help you make good choices.

Chapter 8
Eat This or That?
Food Controversies

Over the past 100 years, scientists have made many exciting discoveries about food. Diseases have been cured with specific vitamins or minerals. We know how many calories are in food. However, we know so much about our food today that most of us are left confused. Do we eat this or that?

And with the prevalence of genetic modifications of food today, things get even more confusing. It feels like the human race is getting farther away from our ancestral roots, when we hunted and gathered our food off the land.

Over the past few years, some big controversies have developed over the safety of eating soy, sugar, salt, meat, wheat, milk and dairy products, and caffeine. Let's review some of these controversies to help us make healthy food decisions.

Is Soy Protein Safe?

A little green soybean that has been enjoyed for thousands of years has caused a lot of confusion and controversy over the past decade. Here are some of the various and sometimes conflicting claims made about soy:

- Soy is good for heart health.
- Soy is good for bone health.
- Soy can increase breast cancer.
- Soy can reduce the risk of colon cancer.

+ Soy is good for reducing menopause symptoms.

+ Soy will disrupt your hormones, causing infertility and promoting breast cancer.

+ Soy causes thyroid problems.

+ Megadoses of soy formula have contributed to premature sexual development in girls.

+ Tofu shrinks your brain and even reduces penis size.

+ Soy is making children gay.

What is causing all this controversy? First, part of the controversy over soy stems from the fact that it is made of isoflavones, a type of phytoestrogen (plant estrogen). The isoflavones in soy have a mild estrogenic effect as compared to the body's natural form of estrogen, estradiol. Not all women get the estrogenic effect from soy, and for those who do, it is minuscule compared to estradiol.

Second, some of the controversy is over soy isolate. The term "isolate" for soybeans means the product has to be at least 90 percent protein—it's soybean minus the fats and the fibrous bean part. Soy isolate is a food ingredient that has been separated, or isolated, from the other components of the soybean, making it 90 percent to 95 percent protein and nearly carbohydrate-free.

Soy protein isolate is used throughout the food industry to boost nutrition and functionality given the cholesterol-free, nearly fat-free, carb-free makeup of the protein source. You can find it in cereals, breads, veggie burgers and deli meat products.

The United States Department of Agriculture (USDA) considers isolated soy protein an *extender* or *binder*, not a *filler*.

So why is soy isolate a bad guy in the press and many best-selling books? Today, Americans are eating a lot of processed soy products that include other not so healthy ingredients including salt and sugar. Is soy isolate guilty by association?

The *Eat Like a Woman* motto is to choose whole foods and limit processed foods. If your diet consists of mostly processed foods, then you have a long list of bad guy ingredients to blame for your bad health.

There are many soy foods made from whole soybean ingredients that do not separate the oil from the bean: tofu, tempeh, miso, tamari, soy yogurt, soy frozen desserts (made from whole soybean milk), soy nutrition bars and soy milk.

According to researchers, soymilk products are very useful for pregnant women. Soymilk products contain vitamin D, so they are helpful for people with limited exposure to the sun or those who are allergic to sunlight, as 90 percent of vitamin D is obtained from exposure to the sun. It is also a good supplement for a meal replacement and known for its antioxidant properties. Soy protein has high levels of glutamine and arginine, the two important amino acids for the formation of new muscle tissue.

There are many soy foods and supplements available—soy bars, shakes, tofu, soy milk, edamame, veggie burgers—so it is no surprise there is confusion about what is healthy and what is not.

Let's review the latest scientific research on soy consumed by humans (not lab rats):

1. **Menopause:** Soy may decrease symptoms of menopause, such as hot flashes, but not as much as estrogen therapy, so the results vary between women. There are studies that claim soy "tablets" do not reduce menopausal hot flashes, and other studies that conclude soy isoflavones significantly reduce hot flashes compared to a placebo. Clearly, the effect of soy on hot flashes varies significantly. Regardless, women who do not notice hot flash relief can still love eating soy for its low-calorie, plant-based protein properties.

2. **Cancer:** More research is needed to determine if soy is beneficial for warding off colorectal cancer. Similarly, there is not enough evidence to know whether soy is protective or harmful for breast cancer, but it is recommended that breast cancer patients avoid soy.

3. **Thyroid:** Clinical studies show that soy products do not cause hypothryoidism, but soy isoflavones may take up some of the iodine that the body would normally use to make thyroid hormone. Soy products may reduce the absorption of medicines used to treat hypothyroidism. Discuss with your practitioner if you have hypothyroidism and are consuming a lot of soy products.

4. **Heart health:** Both the ADA and the FDA confirm that people who eat 25 to 50 grams of soy protein per day can help lower their levels of LDL cholesterol ("bad" cholesterol that can clog blood vessels).

As you can see, the current evidence for most of soy's potential health benefits is conflicting; however, claims that soy contributes to premature sexual development in girls, shrinks your brain, reduces penis size, and can make a person gay are absolutely ridiculous and are not supported by science. What we can safely conclude is that everyone metabolizes it differently, so eating soy may affect people differently.

The bottom line is that soy protein is a plant-based protein that is as digestible as other sources of protein. It contains wonderful nutrients, such as omega-3 fatty acids, fiber and B vitamins. If you are vegetarian or vegan, soy can provide a complete protein serving. If you are looking to reduce calories, soy is a good low-calorie protein source. Purchase your soy products from a good source that does not provide soy products with genetically modified organisms, and buy organic if you can.

But how much is too much? It has been estimated that Asian cultures consume about 10 to 30 milligrams of isoflavones from soy per day in traditional whole-food form. In the United States, with so many soy products on the market, our population is consuming about 80 to 100 milligrams per day. Some soy supplements have as much as 300 milligrams of isoflavones.

The Dietary Guidelines recommend choosing a variety of lean proteins, such as soy products, (including fortified soy beverages) as well as seafood, lean meat and poultry, beans and peas, and unsalted nuts and seeds. At this time there is not enough research for the FDA to make specific isoflavone intake recommendations. That said, the FDA approved the health claim that 25 grams of soy protein may help reduce the risk of heart disease. That equals approximately 50 milligrams of isoflavones.

Is Whey a Good Protein Source?

Whey is the liquid that remains after milk has been curdled and strained. It is used to produce brown cheeses and ricotta, as well as processed foods such as bread and crackers. Whey-derived protein is sold as a nutritional supplement, popular in shakes for bodybuilding. If you are lactose intolerant, whey products should be avoided.

The biggest difference between soy and whey protein is the digestion rate. Whey protein is found in milk and is fast absorbing, meaning it is in your body for a shorter period of time.

Whey can boost general protein intake, and in overweight and obese individuals may assist in long-term maintenance of body weight without energy restriction. It can also strengthen the immune system; improve the general vitality of the body; and stabilize blood sugar levels, leading to reduced hunger, lowered insulin levels and increased fat burn. Since whey protein comes in a powdered form, it is very useful when you need a quick fix of protein—protein bars, shakes or supplements.

I use whey protein powder for shakes, and I eat either soy or whey protein bars, depending on the brand and flavor. The secret, as always, is everything in moderation!

Should Refined Sugar Be Regulated?

Today, many claim that sugar (sucrose) has ruined the health of America. This is because refined sugar does not have any vitamins, minerals, fats or fiber, and everything beneficial is removed during the refining process. In fact, consuming refined sugar depletes the body of B vitamins, causing symptoms of heart palpitations, anxiety, insomnia, indigestion, rashes, difficulty concentrating, chronic fatigue, paranoia and cravings for more sugar. In addition, sugar makes the digestive system acidic, which leaches other vitamins and minerals from the body, particularly calcium from bones and teeth. It also suppresses the immune system and causes an overproduction of digestive enzymes, which puts stress on the pancreas. Sugar also inhibits blood flow and affects aging, contributing to dental issues, increased wrinkles and dry skin. Our sugar obsession can increase the risk for heart disease, cancer, type 2 diabetes and obesity.

Sugar is a type of carbohydrate that is high glycemic. Sugar is not evil, but if abused, it can threaten your health and weight. Unfortunately, sugar is everywhere, including ketchup, mayonnaise, yogurt, pasta sauce, peanut butter and even breads.

Sugar is addictive because it releases an opiate-like substance that activates the brain's reward system. That euphoric effect triggers dopamine, our pleasure reward neurotransmitter.

We are all born with a natural preference for sweetness, which through evolution enabled us to know when fruits and berries were ripe and ready to eat. But our sweet tooth is no longer working to our advantage.

From 1970 through 2000, the daily caloric intake among women ages 20 to 39 jumped from 1,652 to 2,028. Sadly, over this period, the percentage of calories we were getting from healthy fats and protein decreased. On average, we consume 25 pounds more sugar annually than women did during the 1970s. Today, our daily caloric intake from sugar—325 calories on average—comes from sweets such as baked goods, desserts, soda and fruit juices. In the past 100 years, Americans went from consuming 5 pounds of sugar per person per year to almost 150 pounds of sugar per person.

Refined sugar is linked to:

- Hair loss
- Attention deficit disorder (ADD)
- Attention deficit hyperactivity disorder (ADHD)
- Skin irritations
- Metabolic syndrome
- Obesity
- Type 2 diabetes
- Dizziness
- Allergies
- Manic depression
- Cardiovascular disease
- Hypertension
- Hypoglycemia
- Colon and pancreatic cancer

In 1967, high-fructose corn syrup (HFCS), the first scientifically engineered sugar, was created. HFCS is a combination of fructose and glucose. It is a clear, sticky liquid with the consistency of maple syrup that can be cheaper to manufacture and sweeter than natural, cane-derived sugar (1.16 times sweeter). Over the years, HFCS also began replacing the sugar in cereals, granola bars and even flavored yogurt.

In 1970, HFCS accounted for less than 1 percent of all sweeteners consumed in America. By 2000, after countless fat-free products were pumped full of sugar to improve their taste, that figure had risen to 42 percent.

Now, HFCS accounts for half of all sweeteners, and the United States is both the largest producer and consumer of HFCS in the world. HFCS has been acknowledged as one of the villains in the obesity epidemic.

Sugar added to food now accounts for nearly 16 percent of the average American's daily overall food intake. Sweetened soft drinks make up nearly half of that. Americans consume 53 gallons of soft drinks per person every year. A typical 20-ounce soda contains 15 to 18 teaspoons of sugar and upwards of 240 calories. A 64-ounce fountain cola drink could have up to 700 calories. Unfortunately, women who drink sodas do not feel as full as if they had eaten the same calories from solid food and do not compensate by eating less. A 22-year study of 80,000 women found that those who consumed a can a day of a sugary drink had a 75 percent higher risk of gout than women who rarely had such drinks.

There is good news. A diet can contain sugar, specifically fructose found in fruits, veggies, and honey, and still be optimal for health. I always keep local honey in the kitchen. When I have a sugar craving, I enjoy a teaspoon of honey.

Sucrose, glucose and fructose are important carbohydrates referred to as sugars. They all provide the same amount of energy per gram but are processed and used differently throughout the body. Fructose is a sugar found naturally in fruits; glucose is made when your body breaks down starches; and sucrose is abundant in sugar cane, sugar beets, corn and other plants. The safest bet is to get your glucose energy from natural food sources such as fruits and vegetables. This strategy worked for our ancestors before sugary drinks were invented.

The American Heart Association recommends that women get no more than 100 calories a day of added sugar from any source. That's about 6 teaspoons (30 grams) of added sugar, both naturally occurring or added, for women and no more than 9 teaspoons a day for men—yet the average American, including both sexes, currently consumes 22 teaspoons of sugar every day.

With all the confusion about how much or what kind of fructose is best, many have replaced sugar with sweeteners such as stevia, a non-caloric sweetener made from the leaves of a shrub that grows in South and Central America. Stevia is about 300 times sweeter than sugar. Early reports that stevia might cause cancer made the FDA demand more information from manufacturers about its safety. A number of major soft drink companies have begun launching stevia-sweetened beverages, sometimes combining stevia with erythritol, a sugar alcohol. There are no long-term studies of the health effects of stevia, however, so drinkers beware.

Regular consumption of artificial sweeteners and artificially sweetened beverages and foods is linked to obesity, type 2 diabetes, metabolic syndrome and cardiovascular events. Artificial sweeteners also encourage sugar cravings and sugar dependence.

Beware of that colorful rainbow of pink, blue and yellow sweetener packets tempting you with zero-calorie promises…it may be toxic to your health.

Here are some ways to reduce the amount of sugar in your diet:

1. Trade sugar packets for cinnamon.

2. Start drinking black coffee. I slowly weaned myself off café mochas by ordering café latte (coffee with low-fat dairy or soy); then, after a few months, I went cold turkey and now enjoy black coffee.

3. Sweeten with a teaspoon of honey.

4. Enjoy Greek yogurt and berries with some walnuts for dessert.

5. Purchase oatmeal that is not loaded with sugar, then add a teaspoon of brown sugar or cinnamon.

6. On your toast, add a little butter (Dr. Jenkins uses the spray version of *I Can't Believe It's Not Butter,* but I go for real butter the old-fashioned way) and cinnamon—it fills you up and tastes sweet. Note that this tip says *a little* butter, and enjoy it on a whole-wheat piece of toast.

7. If you suffer from blood sugar crashes after exercising, have a protein bar or shake with limited sugar an hour before working out.

Wheat: Innocent Until Proven Guilty

For years, experts have advised us to eat whole-wheat products; now there are claims that wheat contributes to obesity, diabetes, autoimmune disorders, arthritis, heart disease and celiac disease. One best-selling book claims that whole-wheat bread spikes your blood sugar more than table sugar and that wheat has been genetically altered, causing bad health. What do we do with this information?

First, let's look at solid evidence. Whole wheat is loaded with nutrients: iron, zinc, vitamin E, B vitamins and magnesium. Second, the history of wheat parallels the history of chronic disease and obesity across the world. Supermarkets today contain walls of wheat and corn disguised in literally hundreds of thousands of different food-like products or genetically modified foods. Americans now consume about 55 pounds of wheat flour every year.

Today, we eat a different kind of wheat than our ancestors did. Today's wheat was developed to meet the demands of a growing global population, and the man who developed it was awarded the Nobel Prize. While the mass production of wheat has allowed us to feed more people, it has also resulted in producing wheat with increased gluten content, which is far less healthy than its predecessor. Wheat gluten is the natural protein derived from wheat or wheat flour. Some blame this new type of wheat for the rise of gluten intolerance, irritable bowel syndrome, celiac disease and food allergies.

Many who believe that wheat is the demon of disease, and eliminate it with a vengeance, may indeed lose weight, but it is most likely the result of reduced calories after cutting out the desserts and junk foods that include gluten. Heather Magieri, nutrition consultant and spokesperson for the Academy of Nutrition and Dietetics, says, "There's nothing magical about eliminating gluten that results in weight loss. Any of us who eliminate or remove cookies and candies from our diets and replace them with fruits and vegetables is going to feel better."

If you wish to go gluten-free because you want to feel better, get evaluated by your health-care provider to determine if you have celiac disease (an immune reaction to gluten that damages the intestines), a gluten sensitivity or a wheat allergy.

If you decide to eliminate wheat from your diet, enjoy naturally gluten-free grain such as buckwheat or quinoa. Eat a balanced diet with fruits, veggies, lean meat and low-fat dairy.

If you are not suffering from celiac disease, gluten sensitivity or a wheat allergy, you will most likely not benefit from a gluten-free diet. Gluten-free diets can be deficient in fiber, iron, folate, niacin, thiamine, calcium, vitamin B_{12}, phosphorous and zinc. Furthermore, gluten is everywhere. It is used as a thickener in jams, jellies, gravies and instant mashed potatoes; it is used as a filler in drug manufacturing; and it is hidden in "modified food starch."

Remember: everything in moderation is the key to good health.

Eat Meat or Not?

Today, many people are vegetarians (who eat no meat, poultry or fish but will eat other animal products, such as eggs and cheese) or vegans (who avoid all animal-based foods and products) for moral, religious or health reasons. However, our digestive system was designed for eating animal proteins—we, as humans, are omnivores. We hold protein longer in the stomach so it is broken down more efficiently. Plant matter passes through more quickly because it cannot be digested efficiently.

So who is healthier, nonmeat eaters or meat eaters? A panel of 22 experts analyzed 25 diets for the *U.S. News*, rating of the best eating plans overall. They also reviewed the diets specifically in terms of their effectiveness for weight loss, heart health, and diabetes management and prevention.

Of the 25 diets analyzed, the heavily plant-based plans were at the top of this *U.S. News'* lists, but reviewers did not universally embrace absolute meatlessness. The Dietary Approaches to Stop Hypertension (DASH) diet got the number-1 spot, closely followed by the Mayo Clinic Diet and the Mediterranean Diet. These top diets include lean proteins and lots of veggies and fruits. A vegetarian diet was number 10; a vegan diet came in number 14. The Dukan Diet and the Paleo Diet, both high-protein diets, came in last.

A meatless diet's power against heart disease is well-documented. In a 12-year study that compared 6,000 vegetarians and vegans with 5,000 meat-eaters, researchers found that vegans had a 57 percent lower risk of ischemic heart disease—reduced heart pumping due to coronary artery disease, which often leads to heart failure—than the meat eaters. Vegetarians had a 24 percent lower risk.

Studies have also found that vegetarians and vegans did tend to have lower BMIs over nonvegetarians. However, a vegetarian or vegan diet does significantly increase one's risk of certain nutrient deficiencies such as vitamin B_{12}, calcium, iron and zinc—especially in vegans.

Most nutritionists would agree that vegetarianism and veganism are far superior to the typical American regimen, but the healthful choices that work best for you are the ones that actually work for you. The *Eat Like a Woman* plan is similar to the Mediterranean Diet, but it supports our non-meat-eating sisters by incorporating plant-based proteins and combining incomplete proteins for a balanced plan that includes supplementing B_{12}, calcium and zinc.

If you are a meat-eater, enjoy grass-fed beef, as it is lower in calories, contains more healthy omega-3 fats, and has higher levels of antioxidants and more vitamins A and E. Selecting grass-fed beef also supports local businesses and is more ecological. Today, the vast majority of cattle spend about 60 to 120 days in feedlots being fattened up with grains (typically corn and corn byproducts such as husks and cobs, as well as soy and soy hulls) before being slaughtered. Grass-fed cows, on the other hand, live out their entire lives on the grassland.

Eating grass-fed beef or organic free-range chicken, animals that have room to roam and eat their natural diet without being pumped up with antibiotics, begins to mimic the type of protein our ancestors consumed.

Many vegetarians and vegans struggle with weight issues, especially as they get older and hit the menopause transition. A vegetarian diet can be a high-calorie diet (cheese, refried beans, snack bars, nuts, pasta, soy hot dogs), and if your portion sizes are too big, it can be unforgiving. Furthermore, if you consume sweetened beverages, fried foods, snack foods and desserts, it doesn't matter if you are a vegetarian or not—you will gain weight. The basics of achieving and maintaining a healthy weight are the same for vegetarians and non-vegetarians: eat a healthy diet and balance calories eaten with calories burned.

Is Milk Good for You?

Many people in America do not consume dairy milk or dairy products because they believe these products are unhealthy. Many claim that dairy products may contribute to allergies, sinus problems, ear infections, type 1 diabetes and chronic constipation.

There are also an estimated 30 million people in America who are lactose intolerant, which refers to the inability to digest foods that contain lactose, the sugar found in milk and foods made with milk. People who are lactose intolerant cannot digest lactose because their small intestines do not have enough of an enzyme called lactase. Fifty percent of adults are lactose intolerant. If you get diarrhea, nausea, stomach cramps, bloating or gas within a half hour to two hours after eating foods that contain lactose, you may be lactose intolerant. However, keep in mind that lactose intolerance is not the same as having a food allergy. Symptoms of a milk allergy start immediately after drinking milk, and symptoms of lactose intolerance take longer to develop.

Did our Stone Age ancestors drink milk? No. Until animals were domesticated over 10,000 years ago, milk was not part of our diet. Humans naturally stop producing significant amounts of the enzyme needed to properly metabolize lactose between the ages of 2 and 5, or after they have been weaned.

Our bodies weren't made to digest milk on a regular basis. Many scientists today agree that it's better to get the calcium, potassium, protein and fats found in milk products from other food sources, such as whole plant foods—vegetables, fruits, beans, whole grains, nuts, seeds and seaweed.

Milk substitutes fill a dietary void for our vegetarian and vegan sisters, animal advocates, and those with dairy allergies or suffering from high cholesterol. Nondairy milk beverages include soy, almond and coconut milks. Almond milk is high in vitamin E, potassium and magnesium. Soy milk provides protein, and many studies claim it helps lower cholesterol levels.

Teen girls aren't likely to be thinking about their risk for osteoporosis, but maybe they should be. A study published in the *American Journal of Clinical Nutrition* looked at the intake of calcium in the diets of more than 350 teen girls and found that the majority of girls were consuming less than the recommended intake of 1,300 milligrams per day. Peak bone density is reached for most women when they're in their early 20s, and what they are eating in their teen years has an enormous impact on the health of their bones later in life.

In defense of milk, new research compared the average national prices per portion with the nutritional value of various foods per 100 calories, and it revealed that milk is a nutritious food for the money. Milk substitutes can be pricey, sometimes $5 to $6 a gallon compared to $3.50 for regular milk. Other studies concluded that dairy snacks reduced appetite and lunch intake compared with water, with yogurt having the greatest effect on suppressing appetite.

Whether you are a milk lover or not, calcium is important to our bone health, especially women from adolescence to our later years. It is crucial for pregnant women and their infants, and during menopause when significant bone loss takes place. Calcium is lost daily through hair, skin, nails, sweat, urine and feces. This lost calcium must be replaced, or the body will take calcium from the bones to perform other functions.

The following is a list of good sources of calcium:

FOOD SOURCES OF CALCIUM	
Gruyere cheese (3 oz)	860 mg
Mozzarella cheese (3 oz)	621 mg
Cheddar cheese (3 oz)	525 mg
Turnip greens (1 cup, cooked)	492 mg
Collard greens (1 cup, cooked)	357 mg
Yogurt (1 cup)	345 mg
Sesame seeds (1/4 cup)	340 mg

continued on page 116

FOOD SOURCES OF CALCIUM	
Soy milk (fortified, 1 cup)	300 mg
Cow's milk (1 cup)	300 mg
Spinach (1 cup, cooked)	245 mg
Tofu (2/3 cup)	190 mg
Broccoli (1 cup, cooked)	180 mg
Blackstrap molasses (1 tbsp)	137 mg
Almonds (1/4 cup)	92 mg

Salt: Is It Really That Bad?

Americans consume more salt than sugar! Of the 2,600-plus food additives, salt is the one used most often, and sugar comes in second. Salt is a dietary mineral and essential for human life. It is composed of sodium chloride, and it's the sodium part of salt that is important for the body, as the body needs a certain amount of sodium to function properly. When we cry, our tears are salty. Salt can cure, seal, clean, preserve and act as an antiseptic. Salt has no calories. Here are some of the benefits of salt:

* It helps the body absorb potassium.
* It helps maintain the correct concentration of body fluids.
* It is an important part of transmitting electrical impulses in the nerves.
* It helps cells to absorb nutrients.
* The sodium in salt is needed to ensure our muscles and nerves work properly.
* The sodium in salt helps maintain normal blood pressure.

The average adult body contains approximately 250 grams of salt (that is about 4 salt shakers worth of salt). We lose salt through normal bodily functions, so it is important to consume a healthy amount of salt daily. However, high salt intake can increase blood pressure and the risk for heart disease and stroke. Salt may also increase water retention before your period and during pregnancy and menopause. Some nutrition experts claim salt is the single most harmful element in the food supply, even worse than saturated fat and trans fat or food additives and pesticides.

The National Health and Nutrition Examination Survey determined that 88.2 percent of the US population—both female and male—exceeded the less than 2,300 milligrams of salt recommended per day. People suffering from hypertension, diabetes and chronic kidney disease, as well as people older than 51 years of age, have been advised to consume 1,500 milligrams a day or less.

Almost all processed foods, junk food, chips, bacon, cheese, pickles, fast food, meat products and breads have high levels of salt. In fact, recent US studies reveal that 77 percent of a person's salt intake is from processed foods. Throw in the salt we add to food during preparation and eating, and most Americans are over-consuming salt.

Here are some tips for reducing salt:

* Select low-salt or salt-free products.
* Add little to no salt to food at the table.
* Taste food before adding salt.
* Use sodium-free spices.
* Select fresh food over processed food.
* Avoid or use sparingly foods prepared in brine, smoked meats, salty snack items, bouillon cubes, soy sauce and canned soups.
* Season with herbs and spices instead of salt.
* Read product labels. It is shocking how much salt is in frozen diet foods!

Salt in excess can be bad for your health, but in moderation salt has benefits. Aim to stay below the recommended level of 2,300 milligrams a day.

Caffeine, Hormones and Blood Pressure

After water, tea and coffee are the two most commonly consumed beverages on the planet. Coffee is the second-largest worldwide commodity, overshadowed only by crude oil. Black coffee is calorie-free and loaded with antioxidants, flavonoids and other biologically active substances that may be good for health. Green tea, especially the strong variety served in Japan, has received attention for its potential role in protecting against heart disease.

Caffeine, found in coffee and tea, has been consumed since recorded history and has many health benefits when consumed in moderation and without dairy and/or sugar added. Caffeine can:

1. Lower your risk of depression by 20 percent.

2. Give you a more positive outlook on life. A recent study revealed that caffeine consumers were more accurate by up to 70 percent at recognizing positive words than other words. This research suggests that caffeine may stimulate parts of the brain connected to positivity.

3. Stimulate the central nervous system by increasing activity of the brain chemical dopamine, your reward and pleasure center.

> **Warning!** Energy drinks can be loaded with dangerously high levels of caffeine that have allegedly caused death. The FDA cautions users to consult their health-care providers to ensure that they don't have an underlying or undiagnosed medical condition that could worsen by drinking these energy products. As a result of current investigations into the safety of these energy drinks and other caffeinated food products, there may be future FDA regulation. In the meantime, practice common sense and extra caution, and monitor energy drink consumption with your children and teens.

There are sex differences in cardiovascular responses to caffeine due to the role of sex hormones. Males showed greater decreases in heart rate after caffeine administration than females. But females showed greater increases in diastolic blood pressure than males after caffeine. The women also showed greater blood pressure changes than men, but weaker changes in heart rate. These sex differences may be related to sex hormones, as blood pressure responses to caffeine were lower in males when estradiol was high, but higher in females when estradiol was high.

More research on the health benefits of tea and coffee is needed, but one thing is for certain: the addition of cream, sugar, whipped cream and flavorings can turn coffee or tea from a healthful beverage into a not-so-healthful one. For example, a 16-ounce mint mocha chip frappuccino with chocolate whipped cream contains 470 calories. Tucked in this beverage (which is actually closer to a dessert) are 12 grams of saturated fat—nearly a day's worth—and 71 grams of sugar, the equivalent of 17 teaspoons of sugar.

Supplements: Too Much of a Good Thing?

Since the passage of the Dietary Supplement and Health Education Act in 1994, dietary supplement use by American women has increased as our knowledge about the role of nutrients in health has increased. Some of the most popular supplements purchased by women are: calcium, B vitamins, vitamin C, vitamin D, multivitamins/minerals, glucosamine, flaxseed or fish oils, iron, folic acid, and coenzyme Q10.

Americans spend about $9.6 billion a year on supplements, yet there is no clear evidence that multivitamins lower the risk of cancer, heart disease or any other chronic health problem. We take supplements to lose weight and protect our bones, heart and mind. Over a third of us take supplements as insurance because we aren't eating correctly, and many of us take them for disease prevention.

Our bodies require more than 45 vitamins and minerals to maintain good health. The best way to obtain nutritional health is by eating a diet rich in vitamins and minerals; however, taking a daily multivitamin with minerals can be a good option if you are not consuming healthy foods.

At different life stages you may need more of a certain supplement and less of another. Be sure to discuss this with your practitioner. Here are some generally accepted guidelines:

- All women of childbearing age need to take folate, or folic acid, to prevent birth defects.
- Pregnant women may need extra iron.
- Postmenopausal women may need vitamin D to protect bones. (However, beware of menopausal supplements that promise weight loss and hot flash relief; most are selling hope in a bottle that is unregulated by the FDA.)
- People over the age 50, as well as vegans and vegetarians, may need extra vitamin B_{12}. Strict vegetarians, those with cancer, or those with liver or kidney stones have an increased risk for developing vitamin B_{12} deficiency. Problems with balance, fatigue, constipation, numbness in the hands or feet, confusion, and soreness of the mouth or tongue are possible symptoms. A B_{12} deficiency is easily treatable, but it can cause permanent nerve damage if left untreated.

Many experts advocate having a blood test to determine whether or not you have a vitamin or mineral deficiency before beginning a supplement regime. Discuss all supplement choices with your health-care provider because there can be some potentially hazardous herbs that can cause nausea, dizziness, liver damage, diarrhea and kidney damage. The FDA provides dietary supplement alerts and safety information online at www.fda.gov/forconsumers/consumerupdates/ucm153239.htm.

Vitamins and minerals can also affect your health if combined with certain drugs, and many medications deplete your body of essential nutrients. If you have cancer, blood-clotting issues, epilepsy, heart disease, glaucoma, high blood pressure, thyroid problems, diabetes, problems with your immune system or liver problems, talk to your doctor before starting supplements. If you are going to have surgery, be sure to tell your doctor if you are using herbal products.

Supplements are not required to have FDA approval, so they do not go through strict testing to ensure safety and quality. Look for a seal of approval or certification of quality from groups that spot-test supplements, such as the United States Pharmacopeia, NSF International and the Natural Products Association. Always check the expiration date.

Although the benefits of some dietary supplements have been documented, the claims of others may be unproven. If something sounds too good to be true, it usually is. Be a savvy supplement user. Watch out for false statements like these:

+ A quick and effective "cure-all."

+ Can treat or cure diseases.

+ "Totally safe" or has "no side effects."

And be aware that the term *natural* doesn't always mean *safe*. If you do take supplements, follow these safety tips:

+ Consider a supplement combination tailored to your gender and age.

+ Take vitamin D with dinner for better absorption.

+ Watch out for vitamin K; it promotes clotting and can interfere with common heart medicines and blood thinners, such as warfarin (Coumadin).

+ Current and former smokers are advised to avoid multivitamins with lots of beta-carotene or vitamin A. Two studies tied them to an increased risk of lung cancer.

+ For cancer patients, vitamins C and E might reduce the effectiveness of certain types of chemotherapy.

+ When searching for supplements on the web, use the sites of respected organizations rather than doing blind searches.

+ For general information on fraudulent dietary supplements, visit the FDA's website at www.fda.gov/ForConsumers/ProtectYourself/HealthFraud/default.htm.

+ For a list of some of the potentially hazardous dietary supplements marketed to consumers, visit the FDA's list of tainted supplements at www.accessdata.fda.gov/scripts/sda/sdNavigation.cfm?filter&sortColumn=3a&sd=tainted_supplements_cder&displayAll=true.

+ Ask your health-care provider for help in distinguishing between reliable and questionable information.

+ Before making decisions about whether to take a supplement, see your health-care provider or a registered dietitian. They can help you achieve a balance between the foods and nutrients you personally need.

Research on vitamins and minerals continues to reveal health benefits at the proper dose for each sex at each life stage, but remember, dietary supplements cannot replace a healthy diet.

See Appendix B for a chart of food sources of various vitamins and minerals and for common supplement recommendations for specific ailments.

Weight-Loss Medications and Supplements: Are They Safe?

There are several prescription weight-loss medications that have been approved by the FDA to be used while practicing a healthy lifestyle. The most common is phentermine, which is sold under many brand names. It is approved for short-term use. It works as an appetite suppressant and can increase the feeling of fullness after eating. Another type of appetite-suppressant drug, Qsymia, is combined with a seizure and migraine drug that increases the feeling of fullness, making foods taste less appealing.

There is also a weight-loss drug known as orlistat that is a fat-absorption inhibitor. The FDA-approved prescription version is Xenical. Orlistat is also sold over the counter as Alli. Both versions decrease the ability to digest and metabolize fats that are ingested, but there are side effects, such as urgent stools, increased gas and oily stools staining on clothing. This drug inhibits the absorption of nutrients, so you should take a multivitamin. Xenical use can lead to a 5 to 10 percent weight loss when combined with healthy eating and exercise habits. Most of the weight loss happens during the first six months. If you are diabetic, obtain your doctor's approval prior to taking any over-the-counter weight loss medication, including Alli.

Amphetamines are a distinct class of drugs that boost energy and suppress appetite, but chronic use can lead to dependence or addiction. If you have a history of heart disease, high blood pressure or stroke you should not take these drugs.

For the majority of the other FDA-approved weight-loss medications, there are significant side effects and financial costs compared with the 10 to 20 pounds of weight loss you may achieve. For instance, the FDA banned the diet supplement ephedra, also known as ma huang, in 2004 because of the health and heart problems it caused. Bitter orange quickly became popular as an "ephedra-free" product, but combined with caffeine, it can cause high blood pressure and increase heart rate in healthy adults. There is no evidence that bitter orange is any safer than ephedra; in fact, the National Collegiate Athletic Association has banned this substance from educational institutions and the student-athlete.

Unless your doctor recommends that you take one of these medications because you are markedly obese and nothing else is helping with weight loss, commit to a healthy lifestyle with realistic expectations instead. If it took you 10 years to gain 100 pounds, do not expect to lose them in 3 months.

The unregulated weight-loss supplement business is booming, and you should always speak with your health-care provider before using anything, especially if you are pregnant, since some of these products can cause birth defects.

When I went through menopause, my rapid 25-pound weight gain forced me to search for fast-acting remedies. I purchased two different over-the-counter weight-loss products that were loaded with caffeine. They exaggerated my menopause symptoms, and my heartbeat was so fast one afternoon that I thought I was having a heart attack. Needless to say, those weight-loss products worsened my situation and I actually gained weight!

It took being miserable and a loss of self-esteem to open my eyes and acknowledge that good, old-fashioned hard work and commitment was my only option. In 3 months, I lost 25 pounds, and I have kept them off for 8 years.

The table shows common over-the-counter weight-loss treatments and what the research shows about their effectiveness and safety.

HOW SAFE ARE WEIGHT-LOSS SUPPLEMENTS?

Product	Claim	Effectiveness	Side effects
Alli—over-the-counter version of prescription drug orlistat (Xenical)	Decreases absorption of dietary fat	Effective, but weight loss is even more modest than that with Xenical	Loose stools, oily spotting, frequent or hard-to-control bowel movements; reports of rare, but serious liver injury
Bitter orange	Increases energy level; suppresses appetite	Probably ineffective	Similar to ephedra: raised blood pressure and heart rate
Chitosan	Blocks absorption of dietary fat	Probably ineffective	Uncommon but include upset stomach, nausea, gas, increased stool bulk, constipation
Chromium	Decreases appetite; increases calories burned	Probably ineffective	Uncommon but include headache, insomnia, irritability, mood changes, cognitive dysfunction
Conjugated linoleic acid	Reduces body fat	Possibly effective	Upset stomach, nausea, loose stools

Product	Claim	Effectiveness	Side effects
Green tea extract	Decreases appetite; increases calorie and fat metabolism	Insufficient evidence to evaluate	Dizziness, insomnia, agitation, nausea, vomiting, bloating, gas, diarrhea
Guar gum	Blocks absorption of dietary fat; increases feeling of fullness	Possibly ineffective	Abdominal pain, gas, diarrhea
Hoodia	Decreases appetite	Insufficient evidence to evaluate	Insufficient information available

Sources: U.S. Food and Drug Administration, 2011; Natural Medicines Comprehensive Database, 2011.

Health is all about balance and guilty pleasures in moderation. Having a good eating strategy can help you obtain your healthy weight.

Chapter 9
Eating Strategies for a Healthy Weight

Without a strong strategy, creating a healthy lifestyle at any life stage is like trying to row a boat without oars. Just wanting to get to the other side of the river won't get you there without the proper tools.

Anything is possible once you have the desire, some knowledge and a plan. At a recent high school reunion, a classmate said, "You are the only one I know who actually went out into the world and did what you said you were going to do, and more!" This was a very sweet thing to say, but I credit a lot of my drive to get things done to the fact that I was the innocent recipient of survival skills learned as an Air Force brat.

For one thing, I never had time to dillydally, because we moved almost every year. If I wanted or needed something, I had to make it happen fast, before the next transfer. When I was 7, I wanted to take ballet classes after seeing a performance of *The Nutcracker,* so I immediately asked Mom. She always made these types of requests happen, so I was a lucky kid.

During my first ballet class, wearing shiny new black slippers and a scooped-neck leotard with pink tights, I had to figure out how to fit in with the already existing class, not knowing a thing about ballet. The teacher was speaking in French, "Plié, jeté and arabesque." What the heck was she saying? I just tried to do whatever the girl in front of me was doing… heels together, squat down, leg up, arm high, leap across the room. It was fun, although I have no doubt I looked like a klutz in a new leotard with a big smile.

The girls in the class had been taking ballet for the past year. They knew the steps and routines. I wanted to make friends, learn the dances and have fun.

I had the desire but needed the knowledge, so I created a plan. I have used this strategy ever since.

Here's how to get what you want:

+ **Know what you want.** I wanted to learn ballet, a simple goal. As we get older and life gets more complicated, this can be a more difficult task, especially for women.

+ **Ask for help.** It's okay not to know everything. There was no way I was going to fake my way through ballet class.

+ **Find friends with the same desire.** Find others to join your cause; it's a lot more fun being part of a team—and less embarrassing.

+ **Create a plan.** After my first ballet class, I found another girl who did not know any of the steps either, so I invited her to join me and asked for extra help after class.

+ **Include practical steps you can achieve.** I knew it would take more than one make-up class session to catch up. I asked my mom if she could bring me to class earlier so I could get extra practice time before class and focus on the new steps during the actual lesson. We picked up my new friend on the way.

+ **Collect information.** Create a safe, realistic plan so that success is possible. It was going to take months to catch up, so I did not beat myself up comparing myself to others. This rookie was on a mission.

+ **Keep a positive attitude.** Believe that you can do what you are trying to do.

+ **Execute.** If you can see it, you can be it!

I was okay with not knowing the ballet routine because I had a plan with realistic goals. I had fun, made friends, and I used my plan to accomplish my goal. I continued dancing through college until that fateful leap that injured my ankle for life. That was the end of ballet.

Then I created a new plan. Now I love social dancing without all the leaping, and I enjoy ballroom dance classes whenever I have time. Desire, knowledge and a plan are great tools for creating your dreams and experiencing them as they become reality.

This chapter is loaded with strategies to obtain and maintain a healthy weight and tools to set realistic goals.

Meal Timing and Portion Sizes Matter

Our food portions change with each life stage and vary depending on activity level, amount of muscle mass and overall health. How much and when you eat can affect your health and weight.

Meal Timing

A new study recently announced that those who ate a bigger breakfast and smaller dinner lost more weight compared to people who ate a small breakfast and big dinner. The high-calorie breakfast group experienced a 61 percent greater weight loss than the other group. They also had a 35 percent greater reduction in waist circumference and 17 percent greater reduction in body fat.

> People who eat lunch at a computer eat a bigger snack 30 minutes later compared with those who eat without distractions. Put down the mouse and pull up to the dining room table.

For women at a normal to overweight body mass index (BMI), eating three meals, with snacks in between, with breakfast being the highest-calorie meal, is a winning formula, but for obese women, larger meals may prove healthier. Recent research suggests all-day snacking might not be as beneficial as previously thought, especially for obese women. Eating fewer, bigger meals—three balanced meals a day—may be more advantageous metabolically for obese women compared to eating smaller, more frequent meals throughout the day.

More than a third of our population is obese and being coached to consume smaller meals throughout the day. This strategy works for women at a normal to overweight BMI, but this study suggests that obese women would benefit from eating three balanced meals a day, with breakfast being the largest meal to manage cravings.

Portion Sizes Matter

We live in a super-sized society with portions almost doubling in the last 20 years, contributing to the obesity epidemic. Refined grains, added fats and added sugars in larger portions have sabotaged the health of America.

Thinking about portion sizes is a drag, and honestly the only time you need to look at portions and count calories is when you need to lose or gain weight. Once you learn to eat like a woman, you will start managing portion sizes naturally and automatically.

When I went through menopause and gained 25 pounds in 6 months, I started to eat healthier, but I still did not lose weight. I was eating all real foods—no junk or processed food—yet the scale did not budge. I actually put a few pounds on. It was so discouraging to finally start eating like a health nut and see no results. On my quest to solve this problem, I started tracking calories and portion sizes. After just one day of tracking, the answer was revealed. I was actually over-consuming veggies, fruits, nuts, cheeses, salad dressing and lean meats. A whopping 800 extra calories a day in healthy food!

Adjusting portion sizes is an important step to obtaining your healthy weight.

Use these portion size guidelines:

- **Protein:** 4 to 6 ounces, the size and thickness of your palm
- **Carbohydrates:** 1 cup raw, ½ cup cooked (size of your computer mouse), or medium size (size of your fist, wrist to knuckles, or a tennis ball)
- **Fats:** size of your thumb
- **Water:** 6 to 8 ounces per serving
- **Coffee:** less than two cups per day
- **Alcohol:** 1 or fewer servings per day, depending on beverage
- **Fruit:** 1 cup, the size of a baseball

Portion sizes matter. Calories in and out can't be ignored. It is a mathematical equation that can lead you to your healthy weight or send you to the store to buy bigger clothes. If you picked up this book because you need to change your weight, you must do calculations so you can see the areas that need to be modified and set goals for your plan.

Next, you need to calculate your calorie needs and set goals. If you need to lose weight, make a commitment to lose 1 to 2 pounds per week.

Before calculating your daily calorie goal, you have to know how many calories you are currently consuming. An easy way to figure out how many calories you consume per day is to keep a food diary for seven days, counting every calorie. On the seventh day, add up all your daily calorie totals and divide by 7 days, giving you an average daily caloric consumption number.

There are two numbers you need in order to calculate your calorie goals: the number of calories to cut and the number of calories to consume.

Calculate Your Calorie Cuts

First, you need to calculate how many calories you need to *cut* from your diet in order to lose weight. Using this number, you can figure out how many calories you should eat every day. For every pound you want to lose, you need to cut 3,500 calories from your diet per week. So, for example, if you are eating 14,000 calories a week, you'll need to cut that number to 10,500 to lose a pound.

Losing 1 to 2 pounds per week is a healthy goal. If you have more than 10 to 15 pounds to lose, you may lose more than 2 pounds the first few weeks. Be realistic when setting your weight-loss goals. If you have 60 pounds to lose, plan on losing 2 pounds per week. That would take 30 weeks to meet your goal.

For example, say you want to lose 1 pound per week; that equals 3,500 fewer calories per week, or 500 fewer calories per day. You could go to spin class and burn off 350 calories and cut 150 calories in food—that's doable.

How Many Calories Should You Eat per Day?

Now that you know how many calories to cut, you need to calculate how many calories you will actually want to consume each day to reach your goal weight. All you have to do is subtract the number of calories you should *cut* from the total number of calories you *need* per day to maintain your weight. Keep in mind that you should never consume fewer than 1,200 calories a day, or else you risk putting your body into survival mode and *holding on* to calories instead of losing them!

For example, suppose you consume 2,184 calories per day and want to lose 1 pound per week:

$$2,184 \text{ calories} - 500 \text{ calories}$$
$$= 1,684 \text{ calories per day to lose 1 pound per week.}$$

If you wanted to lose 2 pounds per week, you'd aim for 1,184 calories. However, as I mentioned previously, it is unhealthy to consume fewer than 1,200 calories per day, so you would adjust your goal to eat 1,200 calories per day to lose up to 2 pounds per week.

If you decide to be less aggressive and lose 1 pound per week, the plan is to cut 250 calories a day through exercise and eat 250 fewer calories, to cut a total of 500 calories a day. That is a plan anyone can live with! When you create your plan, keep in mind your lifestyle and set reasonable goals for yourself.

Depending on your basal metabolic rate (BMR) and active metabolic rate (sedentary vs. active), here are the *general* calorie recommendations per life stage to maintain a healthy body weight, according to the U.S. Department of Agriculture:

- Women ages 19 to 30 generally need 1,800 to 2,400 calories per day.
- Women ages 31 to 50 need 1,800 to 2,200 calories per day.
- Women over 50 need about 1,600 to 2,200 calories per day.

The *Eat Like a Woman* Food Pyramid: The Winning Formula!

One of the biggest factors contributing to the success of my previous book, *The Menopause Makeover*, was the ratio of foods.

I designed a food pyramid that worked for women going through menopause, but I discovered after receiving letters from women of all ages that the plan worked for each life stage. Menopausal women shared the program with their daughters and mothers and granddaughters, and it worked for them, too!

These food ratios work because they take into account the fundamental differences between men and women.

EAT LIKE A WOMAN FOOD PYRAMID

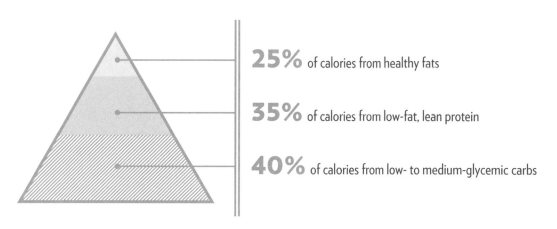

25% of calories from healthy fats

35% of calories from low-fat, lean protein

40% of calories from low- to medium-glycemic carbs

When a woman adjusts her daily intake of carbohydrates, protein and fat according to these recommendations, her healthy target weight will emerge for each life stage. This is very similar to the diets of our Stone Age sisters. According to many experts, these were the average proportions our Stone Age relatives ate:

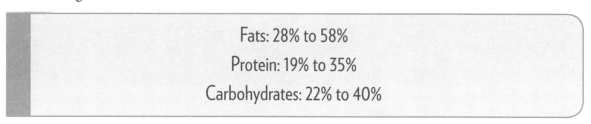

Fats: 28% to 58%

Protein: 19% to 35%

Carbohydrates: 22% to 40%

These ratios are almost identical to the *Eat Like a Woman* Food Pyramid!

Animal protein was naturally much leaner in those days because livestock were not being pumped with hormones and corn feed, so we need to make sure our protein choices are lean today. There were no potato chip trees or Twinkie plants, so natural carbohydrate sources, fruits and vegetables were mostly low to medium glycemic.

Is this food pyramid good for men, too? Yes! But women are designed to hold fat, so these food ratios will help women in particular manage their healthy weight. Men have more muscle mass and can easily eat more carbs and tend not to hold fat as women do.

This food pyramid is perfect for women for each life stage. Most women don't eat enough lean protein and consume too many high-glycemic carbs—our hormones and neurotransmitters will respond positively to lean proteins. Likewise, vegans and vegetarians often don't get enough protein and can easily gain weight. For most women, additional focus needs to go to including healthy proteins in their food plan.

When you combine portion control, meal timing and the *Eat Like a Woman* food ratios, you will start noticing your healthy weight emerge.

Fill more than a third of your plate with lean protein and the rest with low-glycemic carbohydrates. Eat healthy fats—drizzle olive oil over your veggies, not margarine.

Purchase smaller plates. This strategy really helped me *think* I had a full plate of food. Instead of eating on a giant dinner plate that is 11 inches in diameter, find a set of salad plates that are 9 inches in diameter. I often serve my dinner in a salad bowl. It looks like more food, and I do not over-serve the portion.

How Many Grams of Each Food Group Should You Eat?

Here are the latest recommended dietary allowances (RDA):

RECOMMENDED DIETARY ALLOWANCES FOR WOMEN BY AGE RANGE

AGES Life Stage	PROTEIN RDA/grams % of calories	CARBOHYDRATES RDA/grams % of calories	FAT % of calories	FIBER RDA/grams
9–13	34 grams 10%–30%	130 grams 45%–65%	25%–35%	26 grams
14–18	46 grams 10%–30%	130 grams 45%–65%	25%–35%	26 grams
19–30	46 grams 10%–35%	130 grams 45%–65%	20%–35%	25 grams
31–50	46 grams 10%–35%	130 grams 45%–65%	20%–35%	25 grams

AGES Life Stage	PROTEIN RDA/grams % of calories	CARBOHYDRATES RDA/grams % of calories	FAT % of calories	FIBER RDA/grams
51+	46 grams 10%–35%	130 grams 45%–65%	20%–35%	21 grams
Pregnancy	71 grams	170 grams	20%–35%	28 grams
Lactation	71 grams	210 grams	20%–35%	29 grams

Percentages based on "Acceptable Macronutrient Distribution Range" from the U.S. Food and Nutrition Board.

Protein

According to the Institute of Medicine, 0.36 grams of protein per pound of body weight is used to determine protein RDAs. Physically active adults (female and male) require 0.64 to 0.91 grams of protein per pound of body weight each day.

Most women don't get enough protein. Data show that 7.7 percent of adolescent females and about 8 percent of older adult women aren't getting the minimum recommended amount of protein.

Fat

Consume less than 10 percent of calories from saturated fats, and replace solid fats with oils when possible. Eat fewer than 300 milligrams of dietary cholesterol per day.

Carbohydrates

A woman's individualized carbohydrate needs are based on her recommended calorie requirements, weight-management goals and physical activity level. You will note that the carbohydrate acceptable macronutrient distribution range listed in the RDA chart is 5 percent higher than the recommended intake in the *Eat Like a Woman* Food Pyramid. This 5 percent is not going to alter your results toward eating like a woman, but I have found that placing your focus on fewer carbs encourages a slightly higher intake of healthy proteins (plant, fish and animal).

Women are designed to hold carbs and fat for survival, but today our modern lifestyle is less active and food is abundant. A slightly lower intake of carbohydrates can help you maintain a healthy weight. Unless you are an athlete or extremely active, eating like a woman is about balance: healthy protein combined with healthy carbs and healthy fats.

Since carbs are an athlete's primary source of energy during workouts, active women need more carbs than women who are sedentary. Women athletes may require 60 to 70 percent of their calories from carbs per day—this is equivalent to 360 to 420 grams of carbs for a 2,400-calorie meal plan.

Many vegans and vegetarians are not at a healthy weight because this balance is often compromised by eating too many carbohydrates in place of protein—even healthy low- to medium-glycemic choices can pack on the pounds if that is all you are eating. If you are either a vegan or vegetarian and having weight concerns, meet with an expert to discuss modifications so you can honor your eating preference and still make sure you are getting the necessary nutrients to be healthy.

For women ages 19 and older, protein, carbohydrate and fat consumption remain the same. There are variations during pregnancy and lactation, with an increase from 46 grams of protein to 71 grams (about 50 percent more protein), and 130 grams of carbs to 170 to 210 grams (about 30 to 60 percent more). Fat percentages remain the same. Protein is important in each life stage.

Nutrigenomics: The Link Between Genetics and Diet

While we cannot change our genetic make-up, we can influence our genetic expression through personalized nutrition. Incredibly, we can switch genes on and off through nutrition! Nutrigenomics is an emerging field that aims to identify the genetic factors that influence the body's response to diet. It also studies how food affects gene expression.

I had heard of nutrigenomics before but did not truly understand how important it was until my coauthor, Dr. Jenkins, told me about it. I immediately found a local doctor, Dr. Nalini Chilkov, L.Ac., O.M.D., who could order my genetic tests checking for inflammation and hormone issues, both lifelong problematic health areas for me, and interpret the results.

The test was easy; a blood and saliva test. I confess, it was a bit scary thinking about what secrets my genes may be holding, but I was comforted to know that this information can be used to make lifestyle modifications to help offset high-risk genes. For many people, these tests can be lifesaving!

There are 50 genes that play a role in the risk of excess weight gain, with each gene making only a small contribution. The good news is that genes can be altered by lifestyle and environment. Dr. Chilkov says,

> How we live, our everyday choices and environmental exposures, change the expression and activation of the ON and OFF switches of our genes. Factors such as unhealthy food choices, too little exercise, inadequate sleep, and excessive stress damage our genes while healthy nutrient dense organic high-fiber foods, regular moderate activity, 7 to 9 hours sleep each night and regular relaxation and rest promote genes that protect our cells and turn on disease-fighting genes.

Nutrigenomics could hold the key to personalized treatment, but there is skepticism about whether it can truly bring about meaningful modification of the risk factors connected to chronic diseases, due to a lack of large-scale nutrition intervention studies. As the fields related to nutrigenomics advance, and state and federal regulatory guidelines are established, you can discuss this type of personalized diet treatment along with your family history with your health-care practitioner.

My gene test results came in after a week. They confirmed all the things that were wrong with my health: inflammation that put me at cardiovascular disease risk; not metabolizing estrogen normally (a contribution to difficult life stage transitions); and not absorbing vitamin D, folic acid and the B vitamins. I also discovered that I don't metabolize caffeine, and that explains my being able to enjoy a cup of coffee before bedtime and still sleeping like a log. These gene tests are loaded with fascinating information.

The downside is that currently medical insurance does not cover these tests, which are taken only as preventive measure, and all they did was confirm what my doctors and I already knew. I was already taking vitamin D, the B vitamins and hormone therapy, but there were areas that could use additional nutritional support, including an anti-inflammatory diet.

Making Changes: Will or Skill?

Willpower is tested every day—whether it is getting up earlier to work out or choosing an apple over a cupcake at lunchtime. Not having enough willpower was the top reason people cited for being unable to make healthy lifestyle changes, according to a recent survey.

Most people don't always achieve their goals because they struggle with having enough willpower. Willpower is the ability to delay gratification; resisting short-term temptations in order to meet long-term goals. One reason adopting healthy behaviors may be so difficult is that resisting temptation can take a mental toll. Some experts compare willpower to a muscle that can get fatigued from overuse. Fortunately, like a muscle, willpower can be strengthened to help achieve lifestyle-related goals, such as eating healthy or losing weight.

Additionally, individuals need ongoing support to make lifestyle and behavior changes. With the right support, individuals can learn how to make lasting lifestyle and behavior changes, regardless of the importance they place on willpower or the influence of stress.

Willpower is a learned skill, not an inherent trait. It is important to break down unattainable goals into manageable portions. Lifestyle changes are processes that take time and require support. Once you're ready to make a change, the difficult part is committing and following through.

If you feel that a lack of willpower is holding you back from achieving healthy goals, there are techniques that can help you strengthen your self-control.

Here are some tips to make lifestyle changes last:

+ **Share your goals**. Talk about your goals with friends, family or a professional who can help you navigate your feelings and gain skills to successfully change behavior. Being accountable for your actions is very motivating and can help strengthen that willpower muscle.

+ **Start small.** After you've identified realistic short-term and long-term goals, break down your goals into small, manageable steps that are specifically defined and can be measured.

+ **Change one behavior at a time.** Unhealthy behaviors develop over the course of time, so replacing unhealthy behaviors with healthy ones requires time. Many people run into problems when they try to change too much too fast. To improve your success, focus on one goal or change at a time. As new, healthy behaviors become a habit, try to add another goal that works toward the overall change you're striving for.

+ **Be kind to yourself.** There will be days where you don't stick to your plan, but don't give up. Minor missteps on the road to your goals are normal. Resolve to recover and get back on track.

+ **Monitor your behavior toward your goal.** Research shows that people who track their daily food intake are more likely to succeed at weight loss.

Combine these tips with the "how to get what you want" tips on page 125, and take control of your health.

Eating strategies for a healthy weight:

+ Small pieces of food are more filling. Cut up energy-dense foods into smaller pieces.

+ If you want dessert, eat it during your protein-packed breakfast. It will curb sweet cravings for the rest of the day, according to a recent study published.

+ Keep a food journal.

+ Don't skip meals.

+ If you want to lose weight, be persistent. If you have a day full of poor food choices, get back on track during the next meal.

+ Weigh yourself weekly.

+ Eat protein at every meal.

+ Drink a lot of water.

+ Eat brown foods and avoid white foods.

+ Avoid white flour.

+ Focus on healthy habits first and weight-loss goals second.

- Avoid margarine, Crisco or hydrogenated vegetable oils.
- If you need to lose weight, stop eating sugar for the first week so you gain control over cravings and break any addiction to sugar.

Time for Action

The time has finally come to eat like a woman! From personal experience, thinking about changing one thing at a time makes the process so much easier. Not everyone will have weight loss or gain as a goal because this plan for healthy eating works for everyone.

In week 1 of the *Eat Like a Woman* program, you will focus on breakfast only. The foods listed in Chapter 11 represent a collection of food choices that meet the nutritional needs for supporting women's hormonal, neurological and digestive health as described in the previous chapter, with vegetarian and vegan options included. Let's start eating like women!

Chapter 10

Week 1

How to Eat Like a Woman for Breakfast

Supporting good health can be easy once you know the foods that make you feel good and nourish your body for each life stage.

The previous chapters have listed foods for hormone, neurotransmitter and digestive health with variations for each life transition. In week 1, we begin to incorporate those foods into your daily lifestyle, starting with the most important meal of the day—breakfast!

Even though breakfast is a woman's most important meal, consider the following findings:

+ 20 to 40 percent of women skip breakfast.
+ 27 percent of teenage girls skip breakfast daily.
+ 24 percent of women ages 25 to 34 routinely skip breakfast.

Today, with rushed morning routines or trying to cut back on calories early in the day, many women skip breakfast, often only grabbing a cup of java to kick-start the day.

According to statistics and national consumption databases, fewer Americans eat breakfast compared to a generation ago. The most popular reasons for skipping breakfast are as follows:

+ People do not feel hungry after waking up.
+ There is not enough time.
+ It's not convenient.
+ People are not sure what to eat.
+ People forget to eat.

Of women and men who have lost and kept off at least 30 pounds for longer than one year, almost 90 percent reported eating breakfast most days of the week. Breakfast skippers are 4.5 times more likely to be obese than breakfast eaters. Skipping breakfast increases your odds of grabbing junk foods later in the day because brain circuits may be primed toward seeking calorie-rich foods.

Eating breakfast also has the following benefits:

+ Improves memory
+ Reduces the risk of obesity and high cholesterol
+ Decreases insulin resistance
+ Improves strength and endurance
+ Increases intake of essential nutrients that are rarely replenished by other meals
+ Keeps blood sugar levels stable, reducing hunger cravings

Sex differences exist when it comes to skipping breakfast. Females who skip breakfast:

+ Tend to smoke more than women who do not skip breakfast when compared to men
+ Tend to drink more alcohol than men
+ Exercise less than men
+ Tend to intake less iron and vitamin D than men
+ Have a higher incidence of irregular periods than those who do not skip breakfast
+ Show a tendency to suffer from constipation more than men
+ Tend to have a higher serum total cholesterol than men
+ Have a significantly higher incidence of poor self-perception than men

Ladies, breakfast is important to your physical, mental and reproductive health, so do your best not to skip this essential meal.

What If You Don't Wake Up Hungry?

I am a night person and very seldom wake up hungry. I have a cup of coffee and could go all the way to lunch before getting hungry. Does this sound like you? If so, you will have to make an effort to eat within an hour of waking, because breakfast helps to jump-start your metabolism in the morning and fuels your body for the rest of the day.

When you do not eat breakfast, your body enters into a prolonged fasting state. It starts to believe that you won't be eating soon. When you finally eat later in the day, your body stores it as fat because it *thinks*, "I'd better store this for later. I don't know when she is feeding me next."

As discussed earlier, this survival mechanism helped our Stone Age sisters when they often went days without a meal. In our modern world, this can lead to weight gain, fatigue and cranky moods when your blood sugar falls. When you break the fast in the morning, your body can use that food to power you through the day.

Breakfast Basics

Eating a healthy breakfast as your big meal of the day keeps your body fueled so that lunch and dinner can be smaller meals. Less food before sleeping is better, too.

In week 1 you have two missions:

1. Eat breakfast.

2. Eat the right thing for breakfast!

If you think you don't have enough time, schedule it, get up earlier, prepare morning meals in advance and get the whole family involved with your mission. If you are not sure what to eat, this chapter has answers for you. And when you wake up not hungry, set a breakfast alarm on your phone to remind you to eat.

A healthy carb and lean protein breakfast may prevent weight gain by reducing your cravings and suppressing ghrelin. This type of breakfast is also a great brain booster. Since breakfast is the most important meal of the day, your food choices are important. Eating lean protein and healthy carbs—fruits, veggies and whole grains—is a perfect way to start the day.

Where you eat breakfast is important, too. Grabbing a coffee drink and bagel on the go is not only an expensive habit, but also results in you choosing less healthy foods for a quick hunger fix.

When you prepare breakfast at home, you can control serving size, ingredients and calories. When you eat at home, you tend to consume greater quantities of fruits, veggies and whole grains. If you must eat on the go, prepare portable breakfast foods like hard-boiled eggs, fresh fruits, and cartons of Greek yogurt or veggies with peanut butter.

If you want to maintain or achieve your healthy weight, eat breakfast.

If you want to keep those feel-good hormones flowing, eat breakfast.

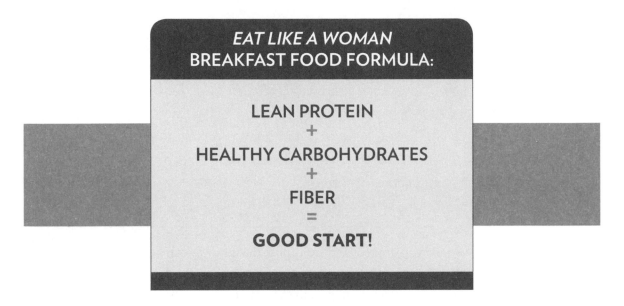

EAT LIKE A WOMAN
BREAKFAST FOOD FORMULA:

LEAN PROTEIN
+
HEALTHY CARBOHYDRATES
+
FIBER
=
GOOD START!

Eat Like a Woman–Approved Breakfast Food Choices

Most people eat the same three or four breakfast choices most of their lives. This week, choose three or four items from this list and only eat those choices. This will establish a routine, so if the morning is busy, you won't grab the wrong foods or no food. If you are already consuming breakfast options on this list, continue to enjoy them or try some new ideas for variety. Many women like a piece of whole-wheat toast in the morning, and adding a hard-boiled egg balances out the meal.

Use the *Eat Like a Woman* master food chart located in Appendix C to select healthy choices or modify your current choices.

Breakfast Options

- Low-fat cottage cheese with berries, coffee or tea (if you like creamers, use a low-fat dairy or non-dairy choice)
- Pre-made protein shake
- Fruit smoothie: blend ½ cup of fruit, 6 ounces of plain Greek yogurt, ¼ cup of uncooked oatmeal, a squirt of honey, and ½ cup of low-fat milk, soy milk or almond milk

For those who like snack bars for breakfast, make sure you purchase a product with higher protein and fiber. Protein fiber bars can assist in reducing the energy intake at the next meal and improve short-term glucose and insulin profiles. When looking at the nutritional label on a protein bar, make sure the grams of protein are close to the grams of carbohydrates. For example, if a bar has 18 grams of carbs and 14 grams of protein, this is a good choice. If the bar has 18 grams of carbs and 2 grams of protein, this is not a high-protein bar. Many high-carb snack bars are marketed as "protein" bars but they actually have a small amount of protein, so check that label.

- Low-fat Greek yogurt with granola and fruit (note that granola can be high in calories, so watch your portion size)
- Whole-grain tortilla wrapped around peanut butter and a banana and served with low-fat milk or soy milk
- Whole-wheat toast with smashed avocado and a hard-boiled egg
- Hot oat-bran cereal mixed with protein powder and served with fruit and low-fat milk or a dairy alternative (cook oatmeal first, then mix in protein powder)
- Whole-wheat pita (I purchase brands that have ½ servings since many whole servings are too big with increased calorie counts) stuffed with low-fat cream cheese or low-fat cottage cheese and sliced fruit
- Planning ahead: whole-grain cereal (at least 3 to 4 grams of fiber per serving) with dried fruit and nuts placed in a sealed bag, with a carton of low-fat Greek yogurt or low-fat milk or dairy alternative
- Whole-grain crackers, string cheese and an apple
- Oatmeal (steel-cut Irish oatmeal is yummy and so good for you) mixed with protein powder, then topped with dried fruit, nuts and a dash of cinnamon
- Whole-wheat toast with your favorite nut butter, topped with a sliced banana, and one cup of low-fat or skim milk
- Whole-wheat English muffin topped with a soy sausage patty (or lean ham) and a slice of low-fat cheese
- 2 ounces of smoked salmon, tomatoes and sliced cucumbers on ½ of a whole-wheat bagel
- Baked Breakfast Frittata (recipe on page 236)

- Toasted sourdough topped with baked ricotta cheese and fruit
- Whole-grain varieties (check ingredients list for the words *whole* or *whole grain* for the first ingredient) of breads, tortillas, crackers, bagels or pita breads, topped or stuffed with your favorite trimming or salmon spread made with low-fat cream cheese, canned salmon and your favorite herbs
- Protein pancakes or waffles (with scoop of protein powder in the mixture before cooking), topped with berries, served with light maple syrup
- Hummus and celery and sliced cold chicken leftovers
- Leftover skinless chicken or turkey on toast, with light mayo, enjoyed with fresh-squeezed juice
- Scrambled egg substitute or eggs with your favorite veggies
- Breakfast burrito or whole-wheat pita made with a corn tortilla, filled with two scrambled eggs, sautéed onions, black beans and salsa
- Poached eggs, ½ cup of berries and whole-wheat toast
- Scrambled eggs with spinach and whole-wheat toast
- French toast with pan-fried apple slices and light maple syrup or real fruit marmalade
- Freezer pops made from a mixture of low-fat yogurt, a splash of low-fat milk or soy milk, mixed with 100 percent fruit juice or whole fruit slices (I love these frozen pops with low-fat Greek yogurt, a splash of almond milk and blueberries)
- Sliced apple and celery with peanut butter
- Boiled egg with gluten-free toast and freshly squeezed juice
- Gluten-free muesli with berries and Greek yogurt
- Vegetables with low-fat dip and a hard-boiled egg

The best juice is fresh squeezed. This makes for an easy fruit serving and a great get-up-and-go morning beverage.

Eggs are no longer taboo! Keep some hard-boiled eggs in the refrigerator so you can enjoy this high-protein food for breakfast or a mid-morning snack. Unless your doctor forbids you from eating eggs, eggs are a great breakfast choice, as they are only about 70 calories, 6 grams of protein, 4 grams of fat and 0 carbs!

- Small tortilla, with a few tablespoons of peanut butter and chopped strawberries, rolled and sliced

- Steamed brown rice with scrambled egg and steamed spinach

- Half bagel, spread with almond or cashew butter instead of cream cheese

- Lean bacon or turkey bacon with a hard-boiled egg (Helpful hint: if you fry up a pound all at once, you can keep it in the refrigerator, and bring it with you in a take-along or other air-tight, microwave-safe container.)

Use this plan with the whole family. Post the *Eat Like a Woman* food chart on the refrigerator and let everyone select their three to four breakfast choices.

How you start the day is a reflection of the commitment you have made to celebrate your health and happiness. If you skip breakfast, a desperately hungry wicked witch could be born before lunch-time, instead of a happy princess skipping through the day with a plan!

Focus on breakfast for week 1

Chapter 11
Step 2
Nourish Healthy Emotions as a Woman

Are your emotions affecting your body? Is your body affecting your emotions? Take this quiz to find out.

YES	NO	
		Do you get cranky when you are hungry?
		When you're feeling blue, do you feel better if you eat something carby or sweet?
		Are you moody during your period?
		Do you cry easily?
		When you feel out of control, would you rather reach for food instead of emotional support?

If you answered yes to at least two of these questions, you are like most women on the mind-body roller-coaster ride.

There is no question that our mind-body connection affects how we feel. With so many sex differences from hormones to neurotransmitters, managing emotional health is very different than a man's journey. As I discussed in Chapter 2, what we think affects our physical health, and our body can influence how we feel. Embracing this delicate balance can make a difference in our life experience.

Stress Can Topple Healthy Choices

If a woman feels happy, her odds of making good food choices, exercising and taking care of herself increase. Making time for relaxation and "me time" is vital. However, with many women balancing a career and family, stress is an active ingredient in daily life—and one that unfortunately contributes to food cravings and weight gain. In Part 1, we learned how stress affects the sexes differently. Stress can sabotage making good food choices for both women and men and increase the risk of disease, but because women process stress very differently than men, managing stress is an important part of healthy living for a woman.

When women experience stress:

- It is difficult to lose weight.
- The risk of heart disease and stroke increase, because blood pressure and cholesterol are affected.
- Sex drive may be reduced.
- Periods may be irregular.
- They may experience migraines, irritable bowel, acid reflux, or back and joint pain.
- They may suffer hair loss.
- Fertility is decreased.
- Their risk of insomnia increases.
- Digestion is compromised.
- They may get acne breakouts.
- They may feel gloomy and tearful.
- They have a hard time concentrating.
- They are constantly irritable and cranky.
- They may feel hopeless.
- Damage can be caused to the immune system, making them more susceptible to infections and viruses.
- The aging process can speed up.
- Brain cells that are bombarded by stress signals have little time to recover and eventually begin to shrink and cut connections to other brain cells. This can lower memory, focus and problem-solving skills.

Before modern times, we were designed to survive—to escape predators or other hostile tribes—so when we sensed danger, our bodies quickly released hormones such as adrenaline into our bloodstream. Our heart rates increased so our attention was focused on the incoming danger. Stress was and still is crucial for survival, but today fleeing from a hungry bear is not a common occurrence. Modern-day stress infiltrates our world with a series of smaller stresses, such as surviving rush-hour traffic.

We all experience stress. When I was my father's caregiver during his final months, I felt and looked 10 years older. Every part of my body felt aged, run down, broken. I have never felt stress at that level before, and it took me a year to rebuild and nourish my health.

Daily stress triggers can include relationships, children, family, finances, work deadlines, traffic, busy schedules and even managing your Facebook page. Our self-esteem and sense of feeling in control can affect how much stress we feel. Marriage has been linked to better health for men but less so with women. Nodding your head "*Yes*, I agree!"? You are not alone.

Chronic stress experienced daily can cause havoc on your overall health and happiness, so it is critical to learn how to manage it. Here are some stress-management tips:

⁘ Identify stress triggers, and resolve relationship issues.

⁘ Try stress-relieving activities, such as yoga, meditation, or tai chi.

⁘ Regular exercise releases endorphins, making you feel better.

⁘ Eat breakfast.

⁘ Schedule fun activities.

⁘ Make time for your friends; support is important.

⁘ Pamper yourself a little bit—take a hot bath, or treat yourself to a manicure or massage.

⁘ Get plenty of rest.

⁘ Sing in the shower, car, church, anywhere—singing relieves stress, according to a new study.

⁘ Slow down and take time in the day for yourself.

⁘ Find a relaxing new hobby.

⁘ Start reading for pleasure, and watch a little less television or take up a hobby.

⁘ Free up your schedule—start saying no to others, and yes to you.

⁘ Make a point of laughing every day.

⁘ Disconnect—don't always answer your cell phone.

⁘ Intimacy with your partner can reduce stress.

Studies have confirmed that people who have more social relationships live longer and increase their odds of successfully managing stress.

Eating certain foods can lower your production of stress hormones. Dark chocolate is rich in free-radical-scavenging phytochemicals called polyphenols that can lower levels of cortisone. Participants in a study who consumed 20 grams (0.7 ounces) of dark chocolate, eating small pieces throughout the day for two weeks, had lower levels of cortisone than those who did not. Ground flaxseed, walnuts (1.3 ounces per day) and pistachios (1.5 ounces per day) can lower stress levels. Drinking chamomile extract reduces anxiety.

Small lifestyle changes can manage stress in big ways.

Women and Depression

Depression affects women two to three times more than men, as discussed in Part 1. Prior to age 13, approximately equal numbers of girls and boys experience depression, but more females than males over age 13 become depressed. The estrogen effects on serotonin can partially explain the sex differences with depression. A large part of our female population is dissatisfied with their body shape and appearance, and this also contributes to depression in women.

Clinical depression is defined as being intensely sad or feeling severe desperation for more than two weeks, with those feelings affecting your daily life. Clinical depression can silently rob your life of joy, happiness and healthy relationships. Depression has been found to increase the risk of developing heart disease and metabolic syndrome.

Depression is a disease caused by very real biological conditions, including neurotransmitter shifts, medical conditions (heart disease, thyroid, sleep disorders, head injury), prescription drugs (antihypertensives, sedatives, steroids, anticonvulsants, analgesics), and alcohol or drug use or withdrawal. If you have a family member who suffers from depression, you may be at a higher risk. Women going through menopause are twice as likely to develop depression than those who are premenopausal. There are also other emotional and environmental causes for depression, including response to loss (divorce, loss of parents, empty nest, loss of youth), as well as changes in relationships, financial instability, overwhelming situations and life circumstances.

Physical illness and certain medications such as sedative and pain medications can produce mood disorders such as depression as well. Alcohol is a depressive substance and can worsen depression, as can increased smoking. A deficiency in folate, vitamins B_6 and B_{12}, and magnesium can contribute to depression.

Symptoms of depression include:

+ Hopelessness
+ Sadness
+ Loss of libido
+ Irritability
+ Feeling desperate
+ Difficulty sleeping
+ Feeling tired
+ Feeling worthless

+ Feeling guilty
+ Overly stressed about weight changes
+ Changes in your appetite
+ Activities that made you happy, no longer do
+ Difficulty concentrating
+ Thoughts of hurting yourself

If you have a history of depression, suffered from bad premenstrual stress or postpartum depression, recently suffered a loss of a loved one, or react poorly to fluctuating hormones, you may be at a higher risk for clinical depression. For those women who have experienced depression once in their lives, between 70 to 80 percent will experience it again.

If you feel that you are clinically depressed, talk to your health-care practitioner about possible treatments. Following are some possible treatments for depression:

+ Pay attention to your moods and keep a journal. This information is useful to determine what is causing your depression.
+ A certain class of antidepressants known as SSRIs (selective serotonin reuptake inhibitors) can help treat depression by increasing the levels of serotonin, norepinephrine, and/or dopamine in the brain. Discuss this option as well as other types of antidepressants with your practitioner.
+ For many, making lifestyle changes can alleviate very mild depression.
+ Psychotherapy can help resolve many issues contributing to your depression.
+ Exercise can make you feel better. When your body secretes serotonin (the feel-good hormone) during aerobic activity, your mood will improve.
+ Eat healthfully and eat throughout the day to avoid blood sugar drops.
+ Omega-3 fats have DHA (docosahexaenoic acid) that can work to ease depression by altering the structure of cell membranes in the brain. Eggs rich in omega-3 fatty acids have been found to reduce the risk for depression. Purslane leaves are high in omega-3 and great in salads or added to veggie dishes.
+ Enjoy green tea. It aids in the release of dopamine, our feel-good neurotransmitter.
+ Avoid sugar. Research has found that eliminating sugar can alleviate depression.

- ◆ Avoid excessive alcohol and caffeine (less than 2 cups daily).
- ◆ Get enough sleep.
- ◆ Join a support group, and surround yourself with friends. Women who have been treated for depression are more likely to find spiritual outlets to help them deal with symptoms of depression.

Often women suffering from depression don't even know it. If someone who loves you suggests you get help for depression, listen. Depression can leave you feeling lethargic, and it can render you unable to properly care for yourself. Do not go through depression alone.

Be aware, though, that some antidepressants can contribute to weight gain as mentioned in Chapter 6.

Mood and Food

What you eat or drink can affect your moods, and your moods can affect what you want to eat. Dietary changes can bring about changes in our brain structure both chemically and physiologically.

Foods can directly influence the neurotransmitter system! Let's start with my favorite mood enhancer—chocolate! Chocolate contains a number of potentially psychoactive chemicals, such as anandamines, which stimulate the brain in the same way as cannabis (marijuana), tyramine and phenylethylamine, which have similar effects as amphetamine, theobromine and caffeine, which act as stimulants.

Before you run to the kitchen for a chocolate bar, a reality check—it takes 2 to 3 grams of phenylethylamine to induce an antidepressant effect, but a 50 gram chocolate bar contains only .0033 milligrams. I still enjoy a little piece of dark chocolate almost daily because it makes me happy.

Diets that banish carbs leave many feeling cranky, angry, tense, and fatigued, reducing the desire to exercise and select healthy foods.

Eating breakfast can improve mood. The *Eat Like a Woman* Week 1 breakfast formula is lean proteins, healthy carbs, and fiber, so it is no surprise this stimulates a good mood and more energy for the day.

A small study from Texas Tech University tested selenium supplementation of 200 milligrams a day for seven weeks and noted improved mild to moderate depression in 16 elderly participants. Oysters, clams, crab, nuts, seeds, lean meats, beans, legumes and low-fat dairy products are rich in selenium.

Omega-3 fatty acids can influence mood, behavior and personality. Omega-3 fatty acids are found in fish, other seafood including algae and krill, some plants, meat, and nut oils. Many foods such as bread, yogurt, orange juice, milk and eggs are oftentimes fortified with omega-3 fatty acids as well.

Your mood can affect your food choices. When you are angry, you may find comfort by impulsive eating. When joyful, you may experience increased hunger because food brings pleasure. When sad or fearful, people often eat less-healthy comfort foods.

As I said, what we eat can affect our mood and how we feel can affect our food choices. The mind and body are connected. So how do you control craving unhealthy foods?

Food Cravings

There are areas in the brain involved with craving and willpower, as well as brain chemicals. The brain chemicals involved with cravings are:

- Dopamine—motivation, drive
- Serotonin—happiness, calming
- GABA—inhibitory, relaxing
- Endorphins—pleasure and painkilling properties

Being a woman predisposes us to cravings because we have a larger limbic area in our brain, increasing the odds that emotions may trigger cravings. When your neurotransmitters are balanced, it can be easier to make healthy choices. Not getting enough sleep, too much stress or alcohol use can contribute to impulse eating and cravings.

It is important to keep your blood sugar stable throughout the day, as it improves self control. Here's how you can manage your brain chemicals to decrease cravings:

- Eat a lean protein-rich meal (plant, fish or poultry).
- Exercise.
- Drink green tea.
- Eat breakfast.
- Meditate.

Developing acceptance-based strategies for coping with cravings can result in lower cravings and reduced consumption, particularly for those who engage in emotional eating. Self-acceptance is a powerful tool for managing cravings. If you are unhealthy and not feeling good about yourself, it is difficult to have self-acceptance. As discussed in Chapter 2, it's a vicious "Her-mood-al cycle"—you crave food, eat too much food, feel crappy about yourself, and then begin all over again. *Eat Like a Woman* step 2 is dedicated to your emotional health to encourage healthy lifestyle choices.

Eating a lower-calorie diet (not lower than 1,200 calories per day) reduces cravings for fats, sweets, and starches whereas cravings for fruits and vegetables increase. Overeating causes you to want to eat more!

Food cravings change during your monthly cycle. High fat/high complex carbohydrates and low-fat/high-protein foods are more strongly desired at and after ovulation. Interestingly the amount of chocolate candy eaten does not differ between cycle phases—whew, good news.

A fascinating study found that smelling an unfamiliar odor reduced cravings for highly desired foods. They tested this theory using green apple, jasmine and water as the smells while in the presence of chocolate. The non-food odor of jasmine significantly reduced chocolate cravings. This strategy could help those with terrible cravings. I personally tested the theory by placing a vase of lilacs and freesias on my desk, and I must confess I had zero cravings. I did not snack or sneak in a sweet treat all day. It's a great idea; enjoy some sweet-smelling flowers in the kitchen or on your desk—they are pretty to look at and may help those cravings.

Emotions and Relationships

A bad relationship can affect all aspects of your life, causing stress that leads to weight changes and emotional frustration. Relationships may be the most significant contributor to good health or poor health, followed by financial security.

Before I met my Prince Charming at age 46, I went through two decades of dating the wrong type of man. In my 20s, I would stop eating when I was stressed out over a guy treating me poorly, then in my 30s, I started reaching for food as emotional comfort, and in my 40s, I figured it out. Unhealthy relationships can affect your health and weight!

Obviously, I am a slow learner when it comes to men, but once I figured out what was going on and made some big changes such as loving myself, I attracted the right guy!

In this section, when I refer to a "relationship," it can be with your partner, parent, sibling, boss, neighbor—anyone you connect with.

Studies prove that women benefit from healthy partner support. It can lower her blood pressure and increase oxytocin levels, making her feel connected.

Relationships are complex, some are healthy and some are not. If you find that most of the people in your life are negative, it's time to shed those negative relationships. Change will happen when you take control and make good decisions.

Nurturing healthy relationships is a lifelong journey for all relationships. Here are some tips for healthy relationships:

* Set realistic expectations.
* Take care of you.
* Be dependable.
* Learn how to fight—fight fair.
* Listen.
* Be flexible.
* Don't criticize.
* Ask for help if you need it.

* Don't gossip.
* Don't hold grudges.
* Don't play the "blame game"; seek a mutual solution.
* Keep your life balanced.
* Exercise, eat healthy and take care of yourself physically.
* Practice patience; building relationships takes time.

If you have a toxic relationship that includes physical or verbal abuse, you can leave. If safety is an issue, ask for support from a trusted person or a professional.

We all want to be loved, but creating healthy relationships takes effort and sometimes involves periods in your life when you are alone. During these transitions, embrace your most important relationship—*you*. Date you. Love you. When you become a complete person who does not search for another to feel whole, you will be on the road to attracting a healthy relationship—whether a girlfriend, parent or spouse. Fulfilling relationships free up your mind to live your dreams.

A few thoughts about sex. For those in a romantic intimate relationship, sex can have benefits other than reproducing a child. We are born sexual beings, to create life from love. If you are in a gratifying relationship but are having issues with sex—too tired, not attracted to your partner, no privacy, growing apart—decide if a sexless relationship is okay for both of you. As we grow older, intimacy may grow into a deeper bond that does not need sexual activity to be complete. If both partners are okay with this, then this is perfectly fine. If one partner is not okay with this arrangement, make time to discuss your feelings or seek personal counseling.

Sex has health benefits! It can:

* Be a cardiovascular sport
* Lower your blood pressure
* Reduce stress
* Curb irritability
* Boost immunity
* Improve heart health

* Increase self-esteem
* Increase oxytocin levels when you have an orgasm
* Decrease some pain
* Build stronger pelvic floor muscles
* Create deeper intimacy

- Make you happier
- Promote good sleep

- Slow aging
- Help minimize incontinence

There will be times in life when you are sexually active and times you are not; times you are in the mood and times you are not. There may be times when you want it, but your libido has declined due to medical or hormonal issues. Sex should not define your life, but it can enrich it when you are in a healthy relationship.

The Power of Zs: Sleep, Lose Weight and Be Happy

One-third of our life is occupied by sleep, yet many of us suffer from sleep deprivation.

A woman's ever-changing body, from her monthly cycle to pregnancy to menopause, can have an effect on sleep due to physical and hormonal changes. Combined with a snoring partner or feeding an infant every few hours or caring for an aging parent who needs assistance using the bathroom in the middle of the night, and women are often not getting the sleep they need to be healthy.

Pregnancy can either increase or decrease sleepiness. Thirty-five to 40 percent of menopausal women report sleep problems as well. When I was menopausal, night sweats had me up every other hour changing my soaking wet PJs.

Not getting enough sleep can contribute to:

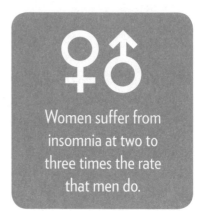

Women suffer from insomnia at two to three times the rate that men do.

- Increased cravings, causing weight gain
- Higher levels of anxiety
- Depression
- Impaired cognition
- Higher risk of stroke and hypertension
- Heart disease

- Increased risk of breast cancer
- Higher risk of diabetes
- Higher risk of injury
- Dreams and emotional responses being affected
- Difficulty focusing

A poll conducted by the National Sleep Foundation found that 60 percent of women get a good night's sleep only a few nights each week, with 46 percent experiencing sleep problems nightly.

That's a lot of women not sleeping! As you may suspect, long-term sleep deprivation effects differ between the sexes. An experiment on 27 healthy volunteers found that restricted sleep affected levels of different hormones more in men than in women.

Long-term sleep deprivation may contribute to obesity because it increases the number of calories consumed the next day. This was especially true of women, who consumed an average of 329 more calories when sleep deprived than when well-rested. By contrast, men consumed just 263 more.

When I am tired, I reach for sugar and caffeine for energy. How about you? Regularly eating an extra 300 calories a day would add up to about 30 pounds of weight gain over the course of a year.

Let's go back and visit our Stone Age sisters, because it is possible that getting less sleep and craving more food has its roots in evolutionary biology. Some experts suggest that our human ancestors slept less during the summer months when people had to eat more to fatten up for the winter. Now we're fattening up, year round, for wintertime that never comes.

Less sleep reduces the amount of physical activity the next day, increases the appetite-stimulating hormones, and leads to overeating to stay awake.

Here are some tips to help you get a good night's sleep:

* Create a sleep schedule, and follow it each night. What time do you naturally get tired? 11pm? 10pm? Then schedule around your natural rhythms.
* Avoid caffeine, nicotine and alcohol right before bed.
* Enjoy decaf tea.
* Do not watch anything that has "light" one hour before going to bed. Avoid laptops, computer monitors, cell phones and handheld video games during the evening hours because they can disrupt the release of the sleep-promoting hormone melatonin.
* Do not watch TV in bed.
* Take a soothing bath or shower before bedtime.
* Your bedroom should be a sleeping sanctuary.
* Clear your mind before you get under the covers.
* Make sure your room is dark.
* Exercise daily. Vigorous exercise should be done during the morning or afternoon.
* Yoga may help promote good sleep.
* Try aromatherapy for relaxation.
* Own a comfortable bed.

If you suffer from chronic insomnia, consider the following and talk to your health-care provider.

+ Keep a sleep diary.

+ Track a typical night.

+ Document what keeps you up at night.

+ How long did it take for you to fall asleep?

+ How long did you sleep in total?

+ How did you feel the next day?

+ Talk to your partner and see if he/she has noticed any differences in your sleeping habits.

+ Discuss any lifestyle changes you've made to improve your sleep.

+ Ask if pregnancy, PMS or perhaps menopause is affecting your sleep.

+ Are there any current medications that could be contributing to your insomnia.

+ What lifestyle changes do you need to make to get better sleep?

+ Are you experiencing more stress?

+ Discuss a strategy to manage your insomnia.

> ♀♂
>
> Many suffering from sleep deprivation ask for sleeping drugs. Zolpidem, the most popular type of sleep drug, has a known sex difference. Women clear zolpidem from the body more slowly than men. Because of this difference, in 2013 the FDA recommended a 5 mg maximum dose for women vs. 10 mg for men–half the amount.

Most experts recommend getting between 7 and 9 hours of sleep per night. If you get only 5 hours per night, then in 1 month you are at least 60 hours in sleep debt. In a year, this pattern creates a sleep debt (2 hours a day x 365 days) of 730 hours or 30 days. That is 1 month of sleep you are missing! Combined with your monthly "Her-mood-al cycle" (see Chapter 2), pregnancy, menopause, or a snoring partner, it is no surprise you may be feeling fatigued, cranky, and craving sweet treats to boost your mood and energy. This vicious cycle can pack on the pounds and affect your overall health.

The Scale: Enemy or Friend?

I have never met an inanimate thing that has caused more pain or joy on a consistent basis than the bathroom scale. The other day, I stepped on the scale and the number was 7 pounds less than the day before. I was in the best mood all day until my husband said the scale was broken and brought home a new one. I did not step on that new scale for 2 weeks for fear my good mood would be ruined and I would feel fat in all my clothes.

Most of us have a love-hate relationship with the scale, but it can be an excellent tool to manage and track your weight. When I go out to dinner and indulge, there is no way I am stepping on that scale the next morning. Why bum myself out? Many can use the scale daily as motivation, and many do better seeing their friendly scale once a week.

Women have a relationship with their scale. This relationship can cause stress, sabotaging healthy efforts. Are you a weigh-a-holic, weighing yourself every day and sometimes many times during the day hoping to see a lower number? Developing a good relationship with the scale is mandatory in a woman's life.

Here are some weigh-in tips:

- Weigh yourself in the morning on an empty stomach.
- It is best not to weigh yourself more than once a week.
- Your body weight can fluctuate between 2 to 5 pounds in 24 hours.
- Weigh yourself at the same time of the day.
- Remember that 8 ounces of water can translate into about 1 pound of weight.
- Weigh yourself naked. Clothes can add up to 8 pounds.
- Due to your period, there could be about 2 to 7 days of the month when your weight is temporarily higher due to water retention, so stay away from the scale during your period.
- Make sure the scale is on a flat surface, not carpet.
- If you eat a lot of sodium, the next day that water retention will increase your weight.
- If you have been sick and dehydrated, you could lose up to 10 pounds, but those pounds usually come back after you are feeling better, eating normal and hydrated.
- Calibrate your scale.
- Digital scales are the best because you can't cheat by lowering the calibration.
- Keep in mind that permanent weight changes take time.

Bottom line: weigh yourself each Friday morning, and skip the week when you are near or on your cycle. People who lose weight are less likely to regain it if they weigh themselves on a regular basis.

Remember, body composition is much more important than body weight. We are all different; healthy for you will be different from healthy for me.

Spirituality and Happiness

Embracing your spirituality can contribute to inner peace and your foundation of happiness. Having a strong sense of who you are and how you want to live your life can pave the way to a lifetime of good health. And it's no surprise that studies show that a person's health is one of the strongest predictors of happiness. Honoring your spirit is just as important as feeding your body and managing your emotions.

Many feel happier embracing spirituality, and happiness can contribute to a stronger immune system, a younger heart, lower blood pressure, and can often help people cope with pain better. Researchers discovered that 40 to 50 percent of a person's capacity for happiness may be genetically predetermined. Fortunately, evidence suggests that even the unhappiest people can learn to be happier. Those who focus their energy on things that give them pleasure tend to be happier. Aristotle once wrote, "Happiness is a state of activity."

There are numerous things you can do to increase happiness that are also included in the stress reduction section. It is no surprise reducing stress increases your chances of feeling happier.

Lifestyle tips on how to feel happier:

- Choose to be happy.
- Be positive.
- Get healthy—make good food choices and exercise.
- Manage stress.
- Laugh.
- If you drink alcohol, drink in moderation.
- Stop smoking.

- Maintain healthy relationships.
- Be grateful.
- Practice forgiveness.
- Engage in activities you enjoy.
- Give back.
- Smile—it increases feel-good hormones.
- Take a walk.
- Spend time in nature.

What you eat can also contribute to feeling happier:

- Bananas can boost serotonin.
- Walnuts and almonds are good for your brain.
- Leafy greens boost energy.

- Cayenne peppers can relieve depression.
- Oats ease depression.
- Drinking water helps reduce stress.

Having good relationships can nourish healthy emotions. Getting enough sleep can curb cravings, anxiety, moodiness, and even depression. Growing your spirit, and practicing gratitude and forgiveness can contribute to happiness. Being happy can give you the freedom to celebrate a woman's journey through each life stage.

Emotional health is just as important as physical health. Elizabeth Gilbert, author of the bestseller *Eat, Pray, Love,* said, "I wanted to explore the art of pleasure in Italy, the art of devotion in India and, in Indonesia, the art of balancing the two."

Life is a balance of the physical and emotional, and only when both are in harmony can your true self emerge.

Spirituality is the one thing in life you can count on—even if you can't see it. A woman's journey is not complete without it.

> Spirituality is the foundation of the mind-body formula.
> Without it, balance is impossible.

Chapter 12

Week 2

*How to Eat Like a Woman
for Lunch and Dinner*

In the United States, most of us eat three substantial meals a day—breakfast, lunch and dinner—with dinner being the biggest meal. However, in many other parts of the world, lunch is the main meal of the day, while dinner is smaller, and it was once that way in America, too.

In earlier times, the midday meal was known as dinner, and it was the largest meal of the day. Workers would rise early, take a break in the early afternoon to eat a large meal with their families, then return to work and finish the day with a light snack before going to bed. This last meal of the day was known as supper, and generally consisted of cold leftovers from the mid-day dinner.

In the past, eating a substantial lunch made sense. Before technology, it was difficult to work and eat without sunlight. Most people's lives revolved around the sun's cycles—rising early and going to bed shortly after sunset.

As the Industrial Revolution took hold in the 1800s and people started moving from the farm to the factory, workers could no longer take a midday break for a large meal. Instead, they began eating a light lunch, pushing dinner to the evening hours after work.

We now know that this shift to the big meal being consumed in the evening has had health consequences. Research has shown that big breakfasts and lunches result in greater weight loss than a big nighttime meal. People who eat at least two-thirds of their calories before dinner will consume less calories for the whole day than people who eat the majority of their calories at night. As Adelle Davis, 1960s nutrition guru, said, "Eat breakfast like a king, lunch like a prince, and dinner like a pauper."

> ## *EAT LIKE A WOMAN* LUNCH AND DINNER FOOD FORMULA
>
> **LEAN PROTEIN (FISH, POULTRY, LIMITED LEAN RED MEAT OR PLANT PROTEIN)**
> +
> **LOW- TO MEDIUM-GLYCEMIC CARBOHYDRATE (SEE THE LIST OF FOODS IN APPENDIX A)**
> +
> **HEALTHY FATS (SEE THE LIST OF FOODS IN APPENDIX A)**
> +
> **MAKING LUNCH BIGGER THAN DINNER**
> =
> **HEALTHY WEIGHT**

Bigger Lunch, Smaller Dinner

There are many benefits of a bigger lunch and smaller dinner/supper:

- Creates more energy throughout the day
- Increases metabolism
- Burns calories
- Supports a smaller nighttime meal so you don't sleep on a heavy load of calories

During Week 2, focus on making lunch larger than dinner. I have started calling lunch *dinner*, and dinner *supper*.

To make life easier, eat your lunch leftovers for dinner/supper. This small change means less cooking, and eating your calories when you need them—during the day. Unfortunately, most eat dinner leftovers for lunch. We have it backward.

Since most of us have more time to prepare a healthy meal at the end of the day, make larger portions so you can eat them for lunch the next day. Or prepare a few dishes on your day off, and place lunch portions in separate containers so you can grab before dashing out for the day. I often prepare a large dish to last throughout the week, place lunch portions into containers, and freeze so I have a stock of prepared healthy meals at hand. It takes preparation, but once you get ahead with a few dishes, it ensures that you are eating enough for lunch and it can save money you would have spent getting fast food.

Taking a break in the middle of the day to eat a major meal is good for stress levels, too. It forces you to stop whatever you are doing that may be causing stress! Slow down and enjoy your meal. In Europe, it is common to see stores close for two hours midday so everyone can enjoy their big meal of the day. I vote for that lifestyle!

Why aren't Americans enjoying lunch as their bigger meal? Once I did research on labor laws, I found the answer and was shocked! According to the United States Department of Labor, each state has different labor laws and requirements for rest and meal periods. Unfortunately, most of the states that honor lunch labor laws allow for only a half hour break after 5 to 6 hours of work, some allow as few as 20 minutes, and one state that honored lunch break laws only applied it to hotel room attendants only.

Puerto Rico has the right idea: 1-hour break after the end of third hour but before the beginning of the sixth consecutive hour worked. Double-time pay is required for work during the meal hour or fraction thereof.

You can check your state's labor laws here: www.dol.gov/whd/state/meal.htm.

And we wonder why Americans are overweight! We don't have enough time to eat a decent meal at lunch, forcing most to grab unhealthy fast food. Until laws change, those who are paid by the hour will most likely have only 20- to 30-minute lunch breaks.

So how do you have a healthy lunch on limited time?

1. Make meals ahead of time, and pack them to go. This strategy saves money and provides healthy meal options while also controlling portion size.

2. If you have only 20 to 30 minutes, sit down (away from your desk) and eat the food you have prepared.

3. Gather a group of employees and take turns preparing a lunch meal. Enjoy friend-time on your lunch break.

4. Use regular-sized plates for lunch and smaller plates for dinner!

So how many calories should you eat for lunch and dinner? Once you calculate your daily calorie needs (see page 128), use this formula to determine how many calories to eat at specific meals.

**EAT LIKE A WOMAN
DAILY CALORIES FORMULA**

BREAKFAST: 35%
LUNCH: 25%
SNACK: 10%
DINNER: 20%
SNACK: 10%

**OVER HALF OF YOUR
DAILY CALORIES ARE
CONSUMED BY MIDDAY.**

Fast Food

Many of us rely on fast food for lunch and dinner because we don't have time to prepare meals ahead of time or it is less expensive. Fortunately, fast food chains and restaurants are adding healthier choices on their menus.

McDonald's has a wonderful grilled-chicken salad. Bring your own low-fat dressing, and this is a perfect meal. They have grilled chicken snack wraps, fruit and walnuts, and apples slices, too.

Many sandwiches can have a high-glycemic index from the bread and condiment choices. Make sure you are getting adequate protein to lower that glycemic load. Load up on veggies for flavor, and select whole-wheat bread or eat only half the bread.

I know people who have gained weight eating too much sushi. It's actually easy when you look at how much white rice and mayo are loaded in a "dynamite sushi roll." Tempura is just another word for fried food! Enjoy edamame, ask for brown rice, and order simple sushi rolls like a California roll. Sashimi is sushi without the rice—and it doesn't get healthier than that.

Here are some tips for healthy eating of fast food:

* Pre-select food options online first. Check calories, sodium content, fat and sugar.
* Watch out for portion sizes. If it is a super-sized product, split it in half and eat it for "supper" later.

- Order grilled, not fried.

- Drink water with your meal.

- Enjoy a salad with grilled chicken and bring your favorite low-fat dressing.

- Watch out for cheese and croutons; those hidden calories can add up fast.

- It is easy to overconsume calories at buffets, too.

- Order veggie burgers.

- Special order sandwiches without mayo, cheese and special sauces.

- Order black beans rather than refried beans and a soft taco over a crispy shell.

- Order a 6–inch sandwich rather a 12-inch sandwich.

- Roast beef, chicken breast and lean ham are healthier choices than bacon, meatballs or high-fat ham.

- Choose whole-grain bread over white bread or huge white-flour "wraps."

- Order brown rice rather than fried rice.

- Steamed or baked tofu is healthier than deep-fried.

- Instead of fried egg rolls, order hot-and-sour or wonton soup.

- Enjoy thin-crust pizza rather than thick-crust or butter-crust with extra cheese.

Make sure you don't let yourself go hungry, because once that blood sugar drops, so does your willpower to make good food choices. Refer to *Eat Like a Woman*–approved fast foods in Appendix E.

Alcohol

As discussed in previous chapters, women should not consume more than one alcoholic beverage per day. If your lifestyle is busy during the day, you may opt for a glass of wine at dinner, your smaller meal, to relax. For those who love the art of pairing wines with food, dinner may once again be the option you choose.

However, have you ever asked yourself why you are drinking alcohol? Do any of these reasons apply?

- To relax
- Sociability
- Like the taste

- Unhappy
- Lonely
- Addicted

- To ease social awkwardness
- Peer pressure

Once you figure out why you are drinking, you can create an environment to manage alcohol intake. The two main reasons that people drink are for the effect and the taste. Most alcohol is high in calories, and when you drink, you have less control over making good food choices. I tend to relax at the end of the day with a glass of red wine. If I schedule exercise at the end of the day, I usually don't have a drink, because I feel better after working out with those feel-good endorphins flowing. After the holidays, if my weight is no longer in the healthy zone, scheduling a workout at the end of the day is a great way to burn calories, ease stress and eliminate the craving for an alcohol-induced relaxation strategy.

Squeezing in Exercise on Your Lunch Break

Many women use their lunch breaks to exercise because it is the only time they have in their busy day. If they do not have enough time to properly nourish themselves midday, however, they will often overeat at dinner, negating the actual benefit of exercising.

If you are fortunate enough to have time to exercise and eat midday, a good solution is to take a half hour walk then enjoy a chicken salad afterward. If you are working out hard at lunch (spin class), it is not wise to eat immediately afterward. Eat a light meal within two hours of exercising.

Eating a full meal before exercising could leave you feeling sluggish or upset your stomach. A little snack, like string cheese or a few almonds, is perfectly fine prior to exercise.

Exercising at the end of the day, followed by a small meal within two hours, honors the *Eat Like a Woman* small-dinner strategy.

Here are tips for *Eat Like a Woman* week 2:

- Focus on making your midday meal bigger than your evening meal.
- Calculate what percentage of calories you need to consume for lunch and dinner. Dinner should be almost half your lunch meal size.
- Discuss this strategy with your family so everyone is on the program.
- Stay hydrated.
- Eat a healthy snack (see the list in Appendix E) between meals so your blood sugar does not drop.
- Use regular-sized plates for lunch and smaller plates for dinner.
- Start calling lunch *dinner,* and dinner *supper*—it's so European. A mind shift will eventually happen when you start associating the midday meal with a larger portion.
- Ask your family and friends to join in creating this new habit; they will benefit, too!

Refer to lunch and dinner food choices, including vegetarian and vegan options, in Appendix E.

Chapter 13
Step 3
SWEAT: Smart Women Exercise All the Time

After feeding your body, embracing your emotions, and honoring your spirit, the *Eat Like a Woman* program comes to life with exercise. Our Stone Age sisters who provided us with the genetic blueprint we still carry had a higher energy expenditure than modern humans. It is estimated that primitive men must have run 10 miles a day carrying the equivalent of 25 pounds while hunting and carrying the kill home. Women did not get off any easier, carrying children, moving camps, finding and hauling vegetables and other foods, and curing meat and hides. That is the kind of exercise regimen built into the human genetic blueprint, but our modern society has almost completely eliminated human movement. Even 100 years ago, we were moving our bodies to survive: saddling up a horse to get somewhere, harvesting food to eat, going to the river for water—we were physically, actively surviving.

Today, with household appliances, cars, planes, computers, grocery stores and clean water in our homes, we are moving our bodies less. Most of us sit at work, sit in traffic, then come home and sit in front of the television. We are sitting most of the day!

Dr. James Levine, who treats obesity at the Mayo Clinic, says, "Sitting all day is killing us." Levine's research shows that a daily trip to the gym, while beneficial, can't undo the damage done from sitting all day.

When you sit all day, the metabolic engines go to sleep, the muscles stop moving, and the heart slows. Then the body's calorie-burning rate plummets to about one calorie per minute—a third of what it would be if you were moving. Fat and cholesterol levels rise, insulin effectiveness drops and the risk of developing diabetes rises. Levine recommends standing up and moving at least 10 minutes every hour when you are sitting. When I am on the phone I always walk around to get out of my office chair. If I am writing all day, I make sure I get away from my computer and out of my chair every hour. Often I just stand up and touch my toes and slowly roll up a few times, go to the bathroom, check the mail or get a bottle of water.

If you are not doing this and instead sitting all day, the risk of being overweight or obese increases. Exercise is the fountain of youth. It is your golden ticket to good health. Since we are no longer focused on survival, we need to find ways to be more active, both physically and emotionally. Step 3 puts the *Eat Like a Woman* program in motion with exercise recommendations and tips for fueling fitness in the modern world.

Smart Women Exercise All the Time!
Let's SWEAT!

Women who actively incorporate exercise live longer; maintain a healthy weight; have lower cholesterol levels and blood pressure; report being happier; have more energy; and can delay or prevent some cancers, diabetes and heart problems. Almost 38 percent of all female deaths in America are the result of cardiovascular disease, making it the number-one killer of women. Lack of physical activity is a major risk factor for heart disease.

Those who add an hour of mild exercise per week or half an hour of moderate exercise have increased levels of heart-healthy HDL, otherwise known as "good cholesterol," and improved levels of LDL, "bad artery-clogging cholesterol." Beneficial effects have also been found to significantly decrease harmful triglycerides for both sexes.

There are 1,440 minutes in every day. Schedule just 30 to 60 of them for physical activity, and you will add years to your life.

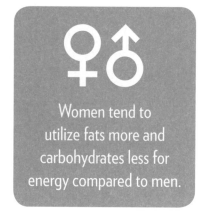

Women tend to utilize fats more and carbohydrates less for energy compared to men.

How Long Should You Exercise?

It is recommended that both sexes exercise for at least 150 minutes per week—that's just 2 hours and 30 minutes. Unfortunately, women are less likely than men to get at least 30 minutes of exercise per day, thereby increasing their risk for heart disease, diabetes and stroke. Women who exercise for at least 150 minutes per week significantly reduce their risk of endometrial cancer, regardless of their body size. If you break it down, 150 minutes per week is doable: 150 minutes is 30 minutes per day for 5 days, or just over 20 minutes per day for 7 days.

An international study revealed that people had health benefits with as little as 75 minutes per week of exercise. That means even exercising for only 15 minutes a day, 5 days a week, can have a measurable impact on health. Of course, more vigorous exercise, as much as 90 minutes per day, further improves health.

An accumulation of 30 minutes of moderate-intensity physical activity throughout the day could be as beneficial as a structured exercise approach. If not having enough time is your excuse not to exercise, try doing 10-minute bouts of movement three times a day. Take the stairs instead of the elevator, push that vacuum with extra vigor, and walk around when talking on the phone—it all adds up!

That said, more is better. Normal-weight people who exercise at a moderate level for at least 150 minutes weekly live about 7.2 years longer on average compared with people who are less active and obese.

How long should *you* exercise? It changes for each life stage, but the overall theme is doing some moderate-intensity activity 30 minutes per day, most days of the week, at the minimum.

Make Time to Exercise

We call it exercise today, but it was survival at our beginnings. I don't know about you, but I hate the word *exercise*—it sounds like a chore, as if you have to do it. I have found activities in my life that get my butt moving, but I don't call them "exercise." I love to dance and swim—both activities our ancestors practiced! I like to bike; a practical way to get around. Yes, I am exercising my body as I move, but I am also having fun.

How many times have you joined a gym and rarely saw the inside of it? If we can't find some fun in "exercise," most of us don't do it, and if we do, it does not last a lifetime. We must create activities in our life that we enjoy. If you are competitive and like to race, then hard-core training could be fun for you. If you are social, perhaps a Zumba class is a good fit for you. If you live a stressful life, perhaps a yoga class is the perfect fit. If you want to keep the family together, playing tennis or a group family sport could be the perfect fit. The sooner you can find an activity you enjoy, the easier it will be to incorporate it into your life.

> The words *activity* or *exercise* both mean a physical activity that is planned for the purpose of conditioning your body.

What's your excuse not to exercise? Too busy? No workout buddy? Too tired? Can't get started even if you want to? Feeling too old? Embarrassed about your body? Feel like learning a new sport or activity is too difficult? Worried it will cost too much money? No place to exercise? Afraid of injury? Already have a painful injury, and activity is painful?

There are many excuses we make to keep from being active, but there are more benefits than excuses. Exercise:

+ Reduces the risk of metabolic syndrome
+ Reduces the risk of depression

- Maintains healthy cholesterol levels
- Reduces the risk of endometrial cancer
- Reduces your appetite
- Can increase insulin sensitivity if you have diabetes
- Can help reverse sarcopenia, a condition associated with inactivity and aging in which fat replaces muscle
- Enables your body to burn calories at a higher rate for between 2 and 24 hours after exercising
- Slows the progression of age-related memory loss
- Lowers the risk of colon cancer
- Reduces the risk of developing coronary heart disease, stroke, and breast and lung cancer
- Primes the brain for learning
- Protects you from chronic stress
- Prevents muscle loss
- Lowers blood pressure
- Increases bone density
- Reduces dementia risk
- Improves your sex life
- Increases strength
- Lowers blood sugar
- Reduces the risk of heart disease
- Helps reduce stroke severity
- Strengthens your heart
- Improves your skin
- Improves digestive function and lowers risk of constipation
- Strengthens lungs
- Reduces the risk of type 2 diabetes
- Strengthens your immune system
- Builds healthy muscles, bones and joints
- Increases your stamina
- Increases general mobility

+ Reduces anxiety and stress

+ Helps you sleep better

+ Can enhance sexual pleasure

+ Increases good cholesterol and decreases bad cholesterol in your blood

+ Improves self-esteem

+ Burns calories, which equals weight loss

+ Strengthens joints and ligaments

+ Helps you look and feel better

+ Makes you healthier and happier

+ Increases your metabolism

If that list of benefits does not awaken the movin' mama in you, perhaps knowing how much exercise fuels your hormones and neurotransmitters will!

Fuel Your Feel-Good Hormones

Activity can increase your feel-good neurotransmitters and hormones as discussed in Part 1. Light to moderate exercise may also have a positive effect on all of the following hormones and neurotransmitters, depending on what type of activity you are doing:

+ **Serotonin** improves self-esteem, relieves depression, promotes and improves sleep, diminishes craving, prevents agitated depression and worrying. Exercise may be the most natural and healthy method of raising serotonin by increasing levels of serotonin's biological precursor, tryptophan.

+ **Dopamine** will stimulate feelings of bliss and pleasure, euphoria, while also helping with appetite control, controlled motor movements, and feeling focused. A deficiency of dopamine can contribute to compulsive eating.

+ **Melatonin** regulates the body's internal clock; it's our "rest and recuperation" and "anti-aging" hormone.

+ **Oxytocin** is stimulated by dopamine and promotes sexual arousal, feelings of emotional attachment, and a desire to cuddle.

+ **Endorphins** elevate and enhance your mood, helping you to feel euphoric, and they are natural painkillers.

- **Norepinephrine** makes you feel happy, alert and motivated. It is an antidepressant, controls appetite, gives you energy and can increase libido.

- Gamma aminobutyric acid (**GABA**) is the anti-stress, anti-anxiety, anti-panic and anti-pain hormone. It leaves you feeling calm, in control and focused. Exercise has widespread effects on GABA. It can restore the balance between opposing forces of activity in the brain and fine-tune the hypothalamic-pituitary-adrenal axis that regulates many body processes.

In addition, exercise is one of the few ways scientists have found to generate new neurons, those cells that process and transmit information through electrical and chemical signals. New neurons are created in the hippocampus, the center of memory and learning in the brain. Exercise exerts its effects on the brain through several mechanisms, including neurogenesis, mood enhancement and endorphin release.

Around age 30, the brain starts to lose nerve tissue. Exercise has a reparative effect on these tissues. So it is no surprise that the best brain function and learning take place during the first hour after exercising!

People who are active can have 5 percent more gray matter in their brain, and that may translate into a lower risk of Alzheimer's disease. The brain benefits from exercise as much as your body.

How Healthy Are You?

Before we start to SWEAT for each life stage, let's determine your level of health now so you can track your progress and select appropriate activities. Once you have your test results, you will be able to set goals to improve your health through exercise. If you are really out of shape, start slowly to avoid injury.

Walking is a great way to test your overall aerobic health. Take this aerobic test and find out how healthy you are. You can take this test using an elliptical or treadmill with computerized distance and time settings, or you can mark off the distance in your neighborhood by driving (note the odometer reading at each mile) and then time yourself walking.

Warm up for 5 minutes, then walk a mile as fast as you can. Use the following scale to gauge your results based on how many minutes it takes you to complete a mile.

Here are some examples of moderate- and high-intensity activities:

Moderate-intensity activities

- Walking briskly (3 mph or more)
- Ballroom dancing
- Tennis, doubles
- Bicycling 5 to 9 mph on flat terrain
- Weight-lifting

High-intensity activities

- Swimming laps
- Aerobic dancing
- Jumping rope
- Tennis, singles

WALKING FITNESS TEST

Age	20–29	30–39	40–49	50–59	60–69	70+
Excellent	<13:12	<13:42	<14:12	<14:42	<15:06	<18:18
Good	13:12–14:06	13:42–14:36	14:12–15:06	14:42–15:36	15:06–16:18	18:18–20:00
Average	14:07–15:06	14:37–15:36	15:07–16:06	15:37–17:00	16:19–17:30	20:01–21:48
Fair	15:07–16:30	15:37–17:00	16:07–17:30	17:01–18:06	17:31–19:12	21:49–24:06
Poor	>16:30	>17:00	>17:30	>18:06	>19:12	>24:06

Now you can take the push-up test to measure your muscular strength and endurance. You will need to time yourself for one full minute, so place a timing device on your exercise mat so you can see it. You can do the push-up in the plank position or the modified (knees bent) push-up position. Place your hands and knees on the floor. Keeping your glutes and abs tight, your back should be in one diagonal line with your head and neck. For the modified push-up your knees are bent, feet should be lifted from the floor and ankles crossed.

Then use the following scale to gauge your results.

MODIFIED PUSH-UPS BASED ON AGE

Age	20–29	30–39	40–49	50–59	60+
Excellent	>48	>39	>34	>29	>19
Good	34–48	25–39	20–34	15–29	5–19
Average	17–33	12–24	8–19	6–14	3–4
Fair	6–16	4–11	3–7	2–5	1–2
Poor	<6	<4	<3	<2	<1

How did you do? If you got a poor score, don't be discouraged. Your body is designed to adapt, so there is no excuse not to incorporate a moderate-intensity activity like brisk walking or ballroom dancing to increase your heart rate and breathing rate. If you got an excellent score, incorporate higher intensity exercises such as spin class or jogging.

If you're very busy, create a time slot for exercise and schedule it. If you are traveling, make time to take a walk, walk the local mall, book a hotel with a gym facility, or pack a jump rope or workout DVD that you can play on your computer in your hotel room. There are lots of YouTube videos for "hotel room workouts" that require nothing but you and some time. If you are afraid of injury, make sure you warm up and cool down, and choose exercises that involve minimal risk. If you don't have the resources to join a gym or attend a class, select activities that require minimal equipment, such as walking, calisthenics, or jogging, or find community programs funded by your tax dollars.

Types of Exercise and Finding an Activity for Life

Finding an activity that you can enjoy is important. We are all different, so not everyone will like the same thing or respond the same way. For instance, I have a friend who loves cleaning her home—it relaxes her and she does it almost every day. She does not go to the gym or formally workout, but she has a normal weight because she is moving every day and not over-consuming food. While cleaning may not sound like your idea of an enjoyable activity, my friend enjoys it, and even though it's not typically thought of as exercise, scrubbing the floors burns 189 calories per half hour for a 150-pound woman. That's more than most women burn walking in an hour.

In fact, in 2013 a research team determined that the time women between the ages 19 to 64 spend doing housework has decreased from 25.7 hours per week in 1965 to only 13.3 hours per week in 2010. They estimated a calorie reduction of about 1,857 calories per week, and that could be a contributor to the obesity epidemic today. However, that said, I am thrilled women's role in society has significantly changed, and we now can make new choices.

If your goal is to lose weight, don't forget to note household chores you do in your calories burned for the day. Do chores and lose weight.

	TOP TEN HOUSEHOLD CHORES FOR BURNING CALORIES (PER ½ HOUR)	
1	Moving furniture	223 calories
2	Mowing the lawn (push, hand)	205 calories
3	Scrubbing floors	189 calories
4	Gardening	167 calories

continued on page 172

	TOP TEN HOUSEHOLD CHORES FOR BURNING CALORIES (PER ½ HOUR)	
5	Washing the car	167 calories
6	Cleaning windows	167 calories
7	Raking leaves	149 calories
8	Vacuuming	129 calories
9	Washing dishes	80 calories
10	Doing laundry	72 calories

Source: Estimations based on a 155-pound person and per 30 minutes of activity. Harvard Heart Letter.

My choice for exercise involves activities other than cleaning. I love short walks with the dogs or taking a spin class. They get me out of the house and calm my mind. Unfortunately, my left ankle injury does not allow me to do impact activities, including long walks. This really bummed me out and I actually got depressed about my new "handicap." Surrounded by good friends who wanted to get me moving again knowing this would make me feel better, I was dragged to a spin class and then a swim class. Both these activities were fun, honored my injury, and kept me healthy and happy.

We are all different, and finding an activity that is enjoyable, fits into your schedule and you can do most days of the week can be life-changing for your health both physically and emotionally. You can find a list of activities with calories burned in Appendix F.

There are three types of exercises you should incorporate in your life: stretching, strength training and cardio.

Cardio at your **target heart rate** can speed up metabolism and burn calories. *Cardio* is the root of *cardiac,* meaning pertaining to the heart, and is adapted from the Latin word *kardia,* which means heart. The following are some of the key benefits of cardio exercise:

+ Relieves stress
+ Improves heart function
+ Reduces risk of heart disease
+ Improves blood cholesterol and triglyceride levels
+ Reduces risk of osteoporosis
+ Improves muscle tone

- Increases production of endorphins
- Reduces risk of diabetes
- Burns calories
- Increases lung capacity
- Improves sleep
- Boosts mood

Intensity through **strength training**—weight bearing and resistance exercises—strengthens muscles and burns fat, increasing lean muscle mass, boosting metabolism and strengthening bones. The following are some of the key benefits of strength training:

- Builds muscle
- Burns calories
- Raises metabolism
- Promotes bone health
- Increases endurance and strength
- Develops anti-aging tissue
- Improves flexibility and coordination
- Improves self-esteem

Stretching adds flexibility, reducing the risk of exercise-related injuries and maintaining joint range of motion so everyday activities are easier. The following are some of the key benefits of stretching:

- Can prevent injury
- Lengthens muscles
- Energizes the body
- Increases joint flexibility
- Increases blood circulation
- Increases flexibility
- Increases performance
- Reduces stress
- Relieves pain
- Enhances muscular coordination
- Improves posture
- Creates a greater sense of well-being

Combing these three types of exercise can increase lean body tissue; decrease body fat; increase bone density; and decrease your risk of coronary heart disease, diabetes, hypertension and even cancer. I notice my skin is clear and I feel better when I exercise. We are all busy women, but creating "me" time is the first step to total health.

EAT LIKE A WOMAN FIT FORMULA

FLEXIBILITY (STRETCH)
+
INTENSITY (STRENGTHEN)
+
TARGET HEART RATE (CARDIO)
=
FIT

**FLEXIBILITY AND INTENSITY
AT YOUR TARGET HEART RATE
EQUALS GOOD FITNESS**

Practice the FIT Formula most days of the week. Start with 2 minutes of warming up, then 8 minutes of stretching to maintain *flexibility*. Add 10 minutes of muscle training, incorporating *intensity* on different muscle groups each day. Next, add 20 to 30 minutes of cardio, at your *target heart rate,* after your strength training or later in the day. This totals 40 to 50 minutes most days of the week, which equals one TV show, the time to pack the kids' lunches (teach them how to make lunch), time to clean up the house in the morning (ask your partner to help, so you can exercise), or time on the phone with a friend (chat while you are power walking). Making time for exercise is possible.

FIT Formula Five-Day Schedule

Flexibility: Warm-up and stretching each day.
Strength Training: Alternate upper and lower body 2 to 3 times a week,
2 to 3 repetitions of 12 to 15. Or focus on one muscle group per day
by doing 2 to 3 repetitions of 12 to 15.
Target Heart Rate: Do 20 to 30 minutes of cardio (60 minutes to lose weight).
See the chart of activities Appendix F.

No more excuses, it is time to SWEAT!

> ## Smart Women Exercise All the Time!
> ## Flexibility + Intensity at your Target heart rate = FIT

See Results with Interval Training

Interval training works the heart, lungs and muscles to the max for short lengths of time. It burns more calories and improves cardiovascular performance. Interval training will improve your strength, speed, agility and stamina.

Interval training works both the aerobic (needing oxygen) and anaerobic (not needing oxygen) systems. When you are pushing yourself to the max during interval training, the anaerobic system uses the energy stored in the muscles for short bursts of activity. Lactic acid is the by-product. During the high intensity part of your interval training, this lactic acid builds, and you enter into oxygen debt. When you recover after the interval, the heart and lungs work together to replace this oxygen debt by breaking down the lactic acid. During this phase of the workout, your aerobic system takes over using oxygen to convert stored carbohydrates into energy.

BEGINNER ROUTINE

1. Warm up 5 minutes at 30% effort.

2. Exercise for 30 seconds at 80% effort.

3. Exercise for 90 seconds at 30% effort.

4. Repeat steps 2 and 3.

5. Finish routine with 15 minutes at 30% effort.

EXPERIENCED ROUTINE

1. Warm up 5 to 10 minutes at 30% effort.

2. Exercise for 30 seconds at 90% effort.

3. Exercise for 60 seconds at 30% effort.

4. Repeat steps 2 and 3.

5. Finish with 5 minutes at 30% effort.

You can use your circuit training routine or cardio routine to do interval training. You can do interval training on a spinning bike, treadmill or the elliptical. Runners incorporate interval training, too.

How do you know what your percentage of effort is? Use your target heart rate. Before beginning interval training, clock a mile at 100 percent effort and note your target heart rate (you will need a heart rate monitor or a monitor on your exercise equipment).

SAFETY TIPS

* Always warm up.
* Start slowly.
* Build the number of repetitions over time.
* Bring your heart rate down during the resting portion of the interval.

You can add variety to your interval training by changing:

* Intensity
* Duration of the work interval
* Duration of the rest interval
* Number of repetitions of each interval

Interval training takes effort and focus. It is easier if someone (trainer, exercise buddy) is timing the intervals and telling you when to speed up and slow down. I prefer doing interval training on the elliptical or spinning bike because I can program the intervals, and focus my energy on performance, not the clock.

Always discuss exercise choices with your health-care provider.

Are You Exercising at Your Target Heart Rate?

Once committed to an exercise regime, your secret weapon is utilizing your target heart rate to ensure an effective workout. The target heart rate is your pulse rate per minute, and it can guide you through safely exercising while maximizing your routine.

Visit EatLikeaWoman.com and go to "health calculators" to find the target heart rate calculator: www.eatlikeawoman.com/toolbox/target-heart-rate.

Wear a heart rate monitor when exercising to track your target heart rate. During cardio sessions, your target heart rate range should be between 60 percent (fitness zone) and 80 percent (aerobic zone) of your maximum heart rate. Monitoring your target heart rate is a great way to make sure you are pushing yourself hard enough to get the fat burning and cardio results you want.

Set goals using your target heart rate. Pace yourself if you have been inactive. If you are not at 60 percent of your target heart rate, push a little harder and watch your fitness level improve. Within six months of regular exercise you may be able to exercise at 80 percent of your maximum heart rate.

Muscle Mass and Sex Differences

Men, in general, have more muscle mass than women because women have more body fat. Muscle burns calories, and because men have more muscle mass, they burn more calories at rest.

Women have 40 to 60 percent less strength than men in their upper body and 25 to 30 percent less in their lower body. Why does this muscle sex difference information matter? Despite a difference in overall amount of muscle mass, we ladies can hold our own for both endurance and strength.

Interestingly, women have a greater resistance to fatigue, the muscle's inability to maintain an expected force, than men. Women are able to sustain continuous and intermittent muscle contractions at low to moderate intensities longer than man.

The differences in muscle mass, exercise intensity, food metabolism and neuromuscular activation have been suggested as contributing factors for the fatigue difference between the sexes. Researchers have shown that women are capable of longer endurance times than men when performing low- to moderate-intensity isometric contractions where a muscle group is tensed against another muscle group or an immovable object, so that the muscles may contract without shortening. This difference is less noticeable when the intensity of the contraction increases above moderate levels.

Keeping our muscle mass tone is important through each life stage. As we get older, women tend to lose muscle and accumulate fat. Research has found that we lose one half pound of muscle every year after the age of 30. That means less muscle to burn calories at rest. When women reach their 40s and struggle with weight gain and complain they can't eat the same amount of food without getting fat, muscle loss is a big contributor.

Estrogen has been shown to influence a difference in burning carbohydrates over fats. During long-endurance exercise, women typically rely less on carbs and more on fat for fuel, while men use more carbs.

Training is not usually a matter of physical boundaries but mental boundaries, 30 percent of training is physical and 70 percent is mental. Determination can change your health profile.

Scientists have shown that it is actually more difficult for women to replace naturally lost muscle as they get older, and this key difference is linked to a key difference in the way men's and women's bodies react to food. It is attributed to hormonal changes during menopause, especially declining estrogen. This exciting discovery stresses the importance that women consume sufficient protein and continue resistance exercise.

Want six-pack abs? It is much easier for men to build strong abs that are defined, because women are designed to hold fat in this area. Having toned abs is possible with a healthy lifestyle, but if you want that defined, hard-ripped look, you will need a strict diet and must train daily. If you are young and maintain your six-pack, it may be easier to keep it as you get older. If you are menopausal and want your first starter-kit six-pack, this may be much more challenging but not impossible. I tried to build my first six-pack in my 50s and after months of hard training and strict diet, I decided that a *toned* tummy was just fine because I enjoy eating desserts and drinking red wine on occasion. Focus on a strong core. And remember it's okay to be soft yet toned.

Keeping your muscle tone will help improve bone density over time, boost your self-esteem, decrease your risk of injury, and give you the strength to do the things you need to do throughout the day.

Recently it has been found there is a difference between women and men in muscle protein synthesis (process the body uses to build muscle). A woman's response to food and exercise declines when she is in her mid to late 60s. Women are at a higher risk for muscle loss because they already tend to have less muscle and more fat than men in early middle age, so when they reach their 50s and 60s, they are already closer to becoming frail.

Injuries

Injuries can happen to anyone at any time. Trained athletes get injuries, too. For many, an injury can develop slowly over time during repetitive movements or from a single traumatic incident. Whether you damage a joint or muscle, knowing how to prevent and how to manage an injury is important. The most common types of injuries are sprains, tendonitis, bursitis and stress fractures, but even a blister can stop you in your tracks.

Injury patterns generally are sport-specific, however, not sex-specific, although there are many exceptions. Women can experience injuries differently than men. Women have a significantly higher risk for injuries to the anterior cruciate ligament (ACL) compared to men. This injury is a tear in one of the knee ligaments that joins the upper leg bone with the lower leg bone— it keeps our knee stable. One obvious reason for the increase in injury to women is our anatomy. Females place more emphasis on their quadriceps muscle than males do, which may partly explain the increased risk of ACL injuries in women. Men may suffer more sprains and strains in the trunk area compared to women, who are more susceptible to lower-extremity injuries from accidents or during resistance training.

Women also tend to land on a flat foot rather than their toes, and have less hip and knee flexion than men do. This can also contribute to the increased injury rate in women. Differences in training, neuromuscular response, and hormonal response may also play a role.

To prevent an ACL injury, try to:

♦ Land safely on the ball of the foot when jumping, and then rock back to the middle to gain balance.

♦ Pivot in a crouched, rather than an upright, position.

♦ Stop gently, using three little steps, rather than one big one.

♦ Do routine exercises to strengthen the legs and keep the knee joint flexible, such as leg presses and squats.

Here are the most common injuries for female athletes:

♦ ACL tears (discussed above)

♦ Concussions

♦ Runners' knee or anterior knee pain syndrome

♦ Stress fractures

♦ Sprained ankle

♦ Meniscus tears (the meniscus is the rubbery, c-shaped disc that cushions the knee and help keep the knee steady)

Among the most significant male/female differences from the point of view of injury is different alignment of the lower body; women have a wider pelvis, their knees are in greater valgus (knock-kneed position), and their feet are more pronated (rolled in); all factors that may contribute to the disproportionate number of knee injuries in women. Women tend to land with their hips and knees straight—causing increased tension on the anterior cruciate ligament (ACL).

The reasons for differences in injury rate are the topic of ongoing research. There are distinct differences between the male and female physique that may be at the base of some of the differences in injury rates. For example, women have more body fat and less lean body mass than men; this is a natural consequence of increased estrogen in women and androgen in men. Although men and women have comparable lower-body strength, females have less upper-body strength, even after undergoing training and adjusting for differences in weight and size.

If you do get injured, think of RICE:

> REST—STOP MOVING
>
> ICE—FOR UP TO 20 MINUTES EVERY HOUR TO REDUCE INFLAMMATION
>
> COMPRESSION—LIMITS SWELLING
>
> ELEVATE—THE INJURED BODY PART

There are several things you can do to prevent injuries:

- Always warm up.
- Stretch.
- Always cool down.
- Wear proper safety equipment.
- Wear proper clothing and shoes.
- Use the correct workout form.
- Take days off.
- Do a variety of activities.
- Start out slowly with less intensity and work up to a longer period of time at a higher intensity.

An injury can affect your life for a short period of time or sometimes for the rest of your life. I had no idea when I sprained my ankle in a dance class in my late teens that it would affect the rest of my life. It took months to heal then 10 years later daily pain entered my life because of osteoarthritis. I share this story with you in hopes that you take all precautions to prevent an injury.

> Research has shown that when people exercise by walking, they walk 30 percent longer if they walk to music.

Honor your body. Our Stone Age sisters had limited activities: walking, running and lifting. Today, we participate in sports and exercise like athletes well into our senior years. Have fun, and do it safely honoring your life stage.

FITNESS FOR EACH LIFE STAGE

STAGE	TYPE OF EXERCISE	HOW OFTEN
Teens	Aerobics—continuous movement of muscles	60 minutes x 3+ days
	Muscle strengthening—make muscles do more work than usual	60 minutes x 3+ days
	Bone strengthening—activities that push on your bones	60 minutes x 3+ days
Reproductive	Aerobics Muscle strengthening Bone strengthening	60 minutes x 3+ days 60 minutes x 3+ days 60 minutes x 3+ days
Pregnancy	Aerobics: moderate intensity	150 minutes per week
	Muscle and bone strengthening	Avoid lifting weights over your head and using weights that strain lower back.
	Avoid activity lying on your back during your second and third trimesters	Do: Swim, walk, dance, Pilates, bike, yoga
	Avoid activities that put you at risk of falling or abdominal injury (i.e. horseback riding, soccer or basketball)	Avoid: Leaping, bouncing, scuba diving, downhill skiing, contact sports, horseback riding
	If you are already doing vigorous-intensity aerobic activity, you may continue provided you stay healthy and discuss how and when the activity should be adjusted over time with your doctor	continued on page 182

STAGE	TYPE OF EXERCISE	HOW OFTEN
Lactation	Aerobics Muscle strengthening Bone strengthening	Begin 4–6 weeks postpartum and with clearance from your doctor. Start with 15 minutes and increase by 2 minutes per day until you get to 45 minutes x 4 to 5 days
Menopause	Moderate aerobics Strength training	30 minutes x 5 days 3 rounds of 8–12 reps, 2x per week
Post-menopause	Moderate-intensity aerobics or vigorous-intensity aerobics Resistance exercises Flexibility Balance exercises	30 minutes x 5 days 20 minutes x 3 days 8 to 10 exercises performed x 2 or more nonconsecutive days 10 minutes x 2 days If needed, to reduce the risk of injury from falls

Sources: The U.S. Department of Health and Human Services, American College of Sports Medicine, American Heart Association.

It's time to start week 3.
Smart Women Exercise All the Time!

Chapter 14
Week 3
*How to Eat Like a Woman
Before and After Exercise*

There are conflicting scientific opinions on whether it is best to eat before exercising. Some say you burn more fat exercising on an empty stomach, but others disagree.

Muscles usually get their energy from carbohydrates, which is why professional athletes eat lots of carb-dense foods before a race or game. If you haven't eaten before exercising, your body doesn't have many carbohydrates in reserve. That forces it to burn fat instead, according to some scientists.

Other experts say that even though people may burn more fat this way, it is mostly fat within the muscles that will be lost and it won't make a big difference to people trying to lose weight.

However, most of these studies were done on young, healthy *men*. Since we are not young, male athletes, *Eat Like a Woman* recommends eating something before exercise. Here's why:

1. Without enough fuel, you won't get the intensity of training you need to get improvements.

2. If your blood sugar is low, you could wind up getting dizzy and you might not be able to exercise as well as if you were well-nourished.

3. Not eating before exercise might make you more prone to injury. Being hungry may lead to weakness, compromising form and increasing your odds of injury.

4. Eating is important so the body has enough nutrients to recover from a bout of exercise.

5. When you postpone breakfast to exercise, it is possible you might eat more afterward.

If you exercise in the morning, get up early enough to eat breakfast—that may mean one to two hours before your workout. Most of the energy you got from dinner the previous night is used up by morning, and your blood sugar may be low. If you don't eat, you may feel sluggish or lightheaded when you exercise. If you plan to exercise within an hour after breakfast, eat a lighter breakfast to raise your blood sugar. Good breakfast options include:

+ Oatmeal with protein powder and fruit
+ Low-fat cottage cheese and fruit
+ Egg white omelet and veggies
+ Protein bar or shake (Protein and carb grams should be similar. For example, 36 grams of carbs and 4 grams of protein is *not* a protein bar.)
+ Hard-boiled egg

If you're not a fan of eating in the morning before you work out, try a protein drink or protein bar. And remember, if you normally have coffee in the morning, a cup before your workout is probably okay. Just don't try any foods or drinks for the first time before a workout, or you risk an upset stomach.

Be careful not to overdo it when it comes to how much you eat before exercise. Here are some general guidelines:

+ **Large meals**: Eat these at least 3 to 4 hours before exercising.
+ **Small meals**: Eat these 2 to 3 hours before exercising.
+ **Small snacks**: Eat these 30 minutes to 1 hour before exercising. An apple with 1 tablespoon of peanut butter or mixed nuts, string cheese, or a 150-calorie protein bar are great options.

Eating too much before you exercise can leave you feeling sluggish or, worse, with a case of diarrhea or stomach cramps. Eating too little may not give you the energy to keep you feeling strong throughout your workout.

I prefer to exercise in the morning and get it off my to-do list. I have a 1/2 cup of coffee with a splash of low-fat almond milk and a 100-calorie protein bar. One hour later, I go to a spin class or hit the elliptical and weights. I have enough energy and strength to do one hour of exercise, and I am not starving afterward.

We are all different, but I have found most women, including myself, do better eating a little something before working out. And don't forget to keep hydrated!

The closer it is to your workout, the less protein you want and the more healthy carbs you want to eat. Eating complex carbs and protein too close to a workout could lead to indigestion, so if you've only got 5 minutes before your workout, keep it simple—grab a few apple slices.

If you are eating a snack before exercising, try to limit it to 100–150 calories. Here are some good snack options:

> Want to lose inches? Weightlifting can burn more body fat than cardio. Pick up dumbbells for faster results. But if you are unable to exercise for long periods or make a full-time commitment, cardio activity may be the most efficient way to lose weight and get healthier.

- Protein shake
- Banana and peanut butter
- Hummus and whole-wheat pita (small, or ½ pita)
- Yogurt and fresh berries
- Low-fat string cheese and a few apple slices
- 100-calorie protein bar
- Low-fat cottage cheese and fresh berries; sprinkle a few sliced almonds on top
- 2 to 4 ounces of sliced chicken with equal amount of baked yams
- Medium apple with a tablespoon of peanut butter
- Hard-boiled egg and whole wheat toast
- Greek yogurt and fresh fruit
- 1 cup of iced coffee and 1 scoop of chocolate whey protein
- 1 scoop of vanilla whey protein powder, 1 cup of orange juice and 1 cup ice, blended
- Low-fat string cheese and carrot

Most of the items on this list work for vegetarians. Here are some that are specifically vegan but can be enjoyed by anyone:

- Edamame
- Plant-based food bars: Raw Revolution, Organic Food Bar, Vega Bars, Pure Organic Bar, MacroBar
- Tablespoon of almond butter with a little granola mixed in and served on a Medjool date
- Medjool dates with almond or coconut butter with crushed cashews and coconut flakes

- Avocado quinoa salad—make quinoa ahead of time then mix in chopped avocado, chopped asparagus, olive oil, vinegar
- Hummus with veggies or pita wedges
- Blueberry smoothie made with soy or almond milk and vegan protein powder
- Trail mix
- Banana and nut butter
- Brown rice cakes with nut butter
- Quinoa with cinnamon and chopped apple
- Soy yogurt with granola
- Raw veggies and black bean dip
- Peanut butter spread over celery (sprinkle some raisins, too)
- Kale chips
- Avocado with salsa rolled in a whole-grain tortilla
- Granola mixed with fruit and milk alternative

Setting Goals

Setting goals drives motivation, and tracking results fuels continued progress. For most, having good exercise intentions may make you feel better but it usually doesn't result in creating lasting change.

> If you write it down, you can make it happen.

Try this goal-setting exercise:

1. Determine your exercise goals. Take into consideration your age, life stage and current weight. Do you need to maintain? Lose weight? Gain weight?

2. Take your measurements, weigh yourself and keep a journal with this information so you can track progress. Weigh yourself only once per week. Take your after measurements once you meet your weight goals.

3. Select the type of exercise. For cardio, do you want to run, walk, play tennis, dance or spin? For strength training, do you want to lift weights or take a yoga class? Choose activities that work for your personality (refer to Appendix F).

4. Pick a time of day to exercise and record it in your calendar.

5. Enroll a buddy to exercise with you.

6. Schedule activities most days of the week.

7. Take a before photo, for your eyes only. This can be depressing, but the payoff will happen when you reach your goal and take the after photo.

8. Make a commitment to you, and decide on a wonderful victory reward once your goal is reached.

Exercise is an important part of a woman's health, yet so many of us don't make time to do it. There are times in my life when I go months without exercising, then it takes great effort to get back on track again. It is so much easier to make it part of your daily life.

There will be good days and days it is impossible to make time for fitness. Finding activities you enjoy increase your odds of success.

The fountain of youth may be an elusive fantasy, but exercise is a major freeway to this destination. In today's modern world, necessary movement has been designed out of our lifestyles.

As you eat like a woman, SWEAT like a woman. Smart women exercise all the time!

See the calories burned per activity listed Appendix F.

3

Eat Like a Woman for Life: Recipes

With the help of my favorite celebrities and world-famous chefs, we have intimate access to healthy and tasty dishes that are mouthwatering.

These *Eat Like a Woman*–approved recipes welcome indulgences, but portion control is key.

Many of these dishes are culinary adventures, while others are delicious inspirations that are easy to make. Push up your sleeves and find your inner chef as you transform your everyday kitchen into a global one. Enjoy these delicious recipes in the *Eat Like a Woman* Food Plans in Appendix D.

Devin Alexander

Devin is a media personality, healthy-comfort-food chef, weight-loss expert, *New York Times* best-selling author and the host of *America's Chefs on Tour* on PBS. Devin loves having a goat cheese and herb omelet with a Devinly Delites™ Muffin for breakfast, a Greek salad with grilled chicken or shrimp for lunch and sushi for dinner. One of her favorite snacks is heirloom tomatoes with a light drizzle of olive oil, plenty of parsley and red onion slivers. Devin's guilty food pleasure is "anything chocolate peanut butter."

Her health advice is, "Don't (ever) diet! If you want to be healthier, make sustainable changes to your lifestyle. Cook for yourself more often."

Helping teenage girls be healthy (both physically and mentally by helping them find their passion) is her passion.

You will love her great-way-to-start-the-day Chocolate-Chip Pancakes, protein-packed Chinese Pepper Steak, fun Tiny Tacos and elegant Honey-Glazed Spiced Pork Tenderloin.

Check out her website at www.devinalexander.com.

CHOCOLATE-CHIP PANCAKES

Aaah, chocolate for breakfast—what could be more heavenly? One of my downfalls has always been warm chocolate-chip cookies. I just love those slightly melty chips! This recipe is my solution to that chocolate-chip craving, guilt-free. These pancakes are chock-full of chocolate chips, so I actually prefer them without butter. But if you like a more buttery taste with just a hint of chips, use only 1 tablespoon of chips and spread 1 teaspoon of light butter over the top of each pancake. You'll add 17 calories and 2 grams of fat per teaspoon. You'll also notice that the recipe calls for very little syrup. Each teaspoon has 17 calories and 0 grams of fat. If you love syrup and want to add more, you can. Just try them first and then add only as little as you possibly can to feel that you're eating a truly decadent meal. Being a true chocolate lover, I prefer them exactly as is.

If you're harried like most of us are, you can double or triple this recipe with great success. The batter will keep in your refrigerator for up to 3 days, which will save time in the mornings.

Please note that pancakes have much more sodium than most people realize. If you get even a half stack at your local pancake house, you're probably eating more than half of your sodium allowance for a day. That said, I usually eat only one or two pancakes for breakfast as a treat to follow an egg white dish instead of eating a big plate of them. You may want to do the same, since pancakes require baking soda and salt to rise, and thus I couldn't reduce the sodium much here.

INGREDIENTS

- 1 egg white, lightly beaten
- $\frac{1}{2}$ cup low-fat buttermilk
- $\frac{1}{2}$ cup whole-grain oat flour
- $\frac{1}{2}$ teaspoon baking soda
- $\frac{1}{4}$ teaspoon vanilla extract
- $\frac{1}{8}$ teaspoon salt
- $1\frac{1}{2}$ tablespoons water
- 2 tablespoons mini chocolate chips
- Butter-flavored cooking spray
- 4 teaspoons pure maple syrup, divided

DIRECTIONS

1. Preheat the oven to 200°F.

2. In a small mixing bowl, whisk together the egg white, buttermilk, flour, baking soda, vanilla and salt. Stir in the water until well-incorporated. Then stir in the chocolate chips and let the batter sit for 10 minutes.

3. Heat a large nonstick skillet over medium-high heat. When a spritz of water causes the skillet to sizzle, working in batches and re-spraying the pan between each batch, pour $\frac{1}{4}$ cup of batter per pancake onto the skillet. Cook them for about 2 minutes until there are bubbles on the top and the bottom is golden brown. Flip the pancake(s) and cook them about another 2 minutes until they are golden brown on the bottom. Transfer the finished pancake(s) to an ovenproof plate, cover with foil, and keep them warm in the oven until they are all cooked. Serve them immediately with 1 teaspoon of syrup per pancake.

CHINESE PEPPER STEAK   MAKES SIX 1-CUP SERVINGS

In addition to loving this dish served hot from the stove, it's become one of my favorites because it makes such excellent leftovers. Toss it on some rice for a complete meal, then save some to reheat in the microwave at work the next day, and your coworkers are sure to be jealous.

Please note: the meat is cooked in batches so it browns properly and ends up being tender.

INGREDIENTS

- $1\frac{1}{2}$ pounds trimmed top round steak, cut into $\frac{1}{2}$-inch-thick strips
- 1 teaspoon black pepper
- $\frac{1}{2}$ teaspoon garlic powder
- $\frac{1}{4}$ teaspoon salt
- $3\frac{1}{2}$ teaspoons extra-virgin olive oil, divided

- $1\frac{1}{2}$ cups sweet onion strips, $\frac{1}{2}$-inch wide, 2 inches long
- $1\frac{1}{4}$ cups green bell pepper strips, $\frac{1}{2}$-inch wide, 2 inches long (about 1 large pepper)
- 1 teaspoon minced fresh garlic
- 2 cups canned crushed tomatoes
- $1\frac{1}{2}$ tablespoons low-sodium soy sauce

DIRECTIONS

1. Place the steak in a medium bowl. Add the black pepper, garlic powder and salt. Toss to season the steak evenly. Let stand for 10 minutes.

2. Place a large nonstick saucepan over high heat. When the pan is hot, put in 1 teaspoon olive oil. Add half of the steak and brown it on all sides, 1 to 2 minutes per side. Remove from the pan. Add another teaspoon of olive oil, then the remaining steak. Brown that on all sides. Remove from the pan. Turn the heat to medium, and then add the remaining 1 $\frac{1}{2}$ teaspoons olive oil, onions, bell peppers and garlic. Cook, stirring occasionally, until just tender, about 5 minutes. Return the steak to the pan, and then stir in the tomatoes and soy sauce. Turn the heat back to high. When the liquid reaches a boil, cover the pan and turn the heat to low. Simmer, stirring occasionally, until the meat is tender enough to fall apart with a fork, about 1 $\frac{1}{2}$ hours. Serve immediately, or refrigerate in an airtight container for up to 3 days.

Recipe taken from Devin Alexander's THE MOST DECADENT DIET EVER! Copyright © 2008 by Devin Alexander published by Broadway Books, a division of Random House Inc. www.devinalexander.com

TINY TACOS

MAKES 10 TINY TACOS, TWO 5-TACO SERVINGS

These miniaturized versions of tacos are one of my all-time favorite, kid-friendly snacks. When Frito-Lay introduced Baked! Scoops, I was so excited that I instantly went to work on creating dishes to fill these little morsels. I just find them so festive. When I conjured these tacos, I couldn't wait to show them to friends and clients. They're so much fun. Not only can you eat 10 of them (how often do you get to eat 10 whole anything—outside this book, anyway—when you're eating healthy?) for only 200 calories. Plus the whole family will be excited to dig into your "diet food." And kids will be more than willing to help prepare them.

INGREDIENTS

- 10 Tostitos Baked! Scoops
- $\frac{1}{4}$ cup finely shredded romaine lettuce
- 2 tablespoons finely chopped tomatoes
- $\frac{1}{2}$ ounce (about 2 $\frac{1}{2}$ tablespoons) finely shredded Cabot's 75% Light Cheddar cheese, or your favorite low-fat cheddar
- 1 teaspoon lower-sodium taco seasoning
- 2 ounces 96% lean ground beef
- 1 tablespoon mild or hot red taco sauce

DIRECTIONS

1. Arrange the Scoops side by side on a plate.

2. Mix the lettuce, tomatoes and cheese in a medium bowl until well-combined. Divide evenly among the Scoops (about 1 1/2 teaspoons per Scoop).

3. Stir 2 teaspoons water into the taco seasoning in a small bowl until it has no lumps. Set aside.

4. Preheat a small nonstick skillet over medium-high heat. Add the beef. Use a wooden spoon to coarsely crumble the meat as it cooks. When the beef is no longer pink, after 1 to 2 minutes, stir in the seasoning mixture. When no liquid remains, after about 1 minute, remove from the heat.

5. Divide the meat evenly among the Scoops, atop the lettuce mixture (about 1 teaspoon in each). Dollop the top of each with taco sauce. Serve immediately.

HONEY-GLAZED SPICED PORK TENDERLOIN   MAKES 4 SERVINGS

I love entertaining with pork tenderloin. As long as my guests aren't averse to eating pork, it's usually one of my first choices. For years, every time I made dinner for a boyfriend's mother, I would butterfly a pork tenderloin and stuff it with goat cheese and sun-dried tomatoes. Then, in *The Biggest Loser Cookbook*, I made a Sweet and Spicy Pork Tenderloin that I started serving to guests often. I later found out that one of the producers served it to the other producers when he had them all over for dinner one night. Now here's another elegant recipe that I love, and I bet you (and your guests!) will too.

INGREDIENTS

- 2 teaspoons paprika
- 1/2 teaspoon salt
- 1 teaspoon freshly ground black pepper
- 1/4 teaspoon onion powder
- 1/8 teaspoon chili powder
- 1/8 teaspoon cayenne
- 1 1/4 pounds trimmed pork tenderloin
- 1 teaspoon extra-virgin olive oil
- 1 tablespoon plus 1 teaspoon honey
- 1 tablespoon minced fresh garlic
- Olive oil cooking spray

DIRECTIONS

1. Preheat the oven to 350°F.

2. Use a fork to mix the paprika, salt, black pepper, onion powder, chili powder and cayenne in a small bowl.

3. Rub the tenderloin evenly with the olive oil. Then rub the spice mixture evenly over it until the tenderloin is thoroughly coated. Cover loosely with plastic wrap and let stand for 15 minutes.

4. Meanwhile, whisk the honey and garlic in a small bowl.

5. Place a large nonstick skillet over medium-high heat. When the skillet is hot, lightly mist it with spray. Cook the tenderloin for 1 to 2 minutes per side, or until just browned on all sides.

6. Place the tenderloin in a roasting pan or ovenproof skillet. (If one end is much thinner than the other, tuck it under to create a similar thickness throughout.) Use a pastry or basting brush to evenly coat the tenderloin with the honey mixture. Roast, uncovered, for 16 to 18 minutes, or until it is just barely pink inside or a meat thermometer inserted in the center reaches 155°F (the temperature will rise another 5°F while standing).

7. Remove from the oven, loosely cover the tenderloin (not the whole pan) with foil, and let stand for 10 minutes. Transfer the tenderloin to a cutting board. Holding your knife at a 45° angle, slice the tenderloin into thin slices. Serve immediately.

Recipe taken from Devin Alexander's THE MOST DECADENT DIET EVER! Copyright © 2008 by Devin Alexander published by Broadway Books, a division of Random House Inc. www.devinalexander.com

Nancy Cartwright

Nancy is an actress, comedian, voice-over artist, Emmy Award winner for being Bart Simpson's voice on *The Simpsons*, author of *My Life as a 10-Year-Old Boy*, philanthropist, and founder of the nonprofit Happy House, Inc. (http://happyhouse.org/site).

Nancy has been my buddy since our final teen years at UCLA. I have always been proud to tell friends, "I know Bart Simpson." It's ironic that troublemaker Bart Simpson is really a girl who lives a clean life and radiates health.

When asked to contribute a recipe for *Eat Like a Woman*, Nancy said, "I am possibly *the worst cook in the world.* If my family finds me cooking, I have given them permission to throw spit wads at me! I cook very little. In fact, a couple of years ago, my housekeeper brought in something she cooked and I promoted her on the spot. That said, I make a *mean* Tortilla Soup that is called just that."

Nancy may not claim to be a cook, but every meal I have eaten at her home is delicious and healthy. For more information on Nancy, visit her website at: http://nancycartwright.com/wp.

NANCY'S MEAN TORTILLA SOUP

MAKES 8 SERVINGS

INGREDIENTS

- 1 tablespoon vegetable oil
- 1 large onion
- 1 tablespoon ground cumin
- One 28-ounce can fire-roasted diced tomatoes
- Two 4-ounce cans diced green chili peppers
- Two 14-ounce cans reduced-sodium chicken broth
- 4 cups cooked chicken, chopped
- One 10-ounce package frozen sweet whole-kernel corn (optional)

- Salt (to taste)
- Freshly ground black pepper (to taste)
- 2 cups corn tortilla strips/chips

TOPPING OPTIONS:

- Shredded Monterey Jack cheese
- Lime wedges
- Fresh cilantro
- Low-fat sour cream
- Hot pepper sauce

DIRECTIONS

1. In a large Dutch oven or deep-dish pot, heat oil. Cook the onion and cumin in the oil until tender, stirring frequently. While the onion is cooking, open the cans of tomatoes and green chilies. By the time you are done, the onions will be tender.

2. Add the broth, undrained tomatoes, chicken, corn (optional) and undrained chili peppers.

3. Bring to a boil and reduce the heat. Simmer, covered, for 15 minutes.

4. You have just enough time to set out any condiments or garnishes (shredded Monterey Jack cheese, lime wedges, fresh cilantro, low-fat sour cream and even hot pepper sauce) and set the table.

5. Don't forget a big ladle—you're going to want seconds.

6. Season to taste with salt and ground black pepper. You can continue to simmer the soup longer if you want. This will tenderize the chicken and meld flavors even more, and make your house smell yummy.

7. Ladle into bowls, top with tortilla strips and thoroughly enjoy!

If you like, you can make this a stew by reducing the amount of chicken broth and adding more chicken, tomatoes and chilies. I like it as a soup.

Zendaya Coleman

Zendaya is an actress, singer, dancer and the author of *Between U and Me*. Our youngest *Eat Like a Woman* recipe contributor is still a teenager, but this girl has hit it big already—she does it all.

Many know Zendaya from Disney Channel's popular TV series, *Shake It Up!*, but I know her as the incredibly graceful "looks like a pro" finalist from *Dancing with the Stars*.

This recipe is low in calories and easy to make—perfect for a quick meal that's loaded with good nutrients honoring the *Eat Like a Woman* food pyramid. Teens need protein and zinc, and the chicken breast in Zendaya's recipe provides 6 percent of a female teen's daily zinc requirements and one serving of protein. You can visit Zendaya's website at www.Zendaya.com.

SHAKE IT UP RICE SALAD WITH GRILLED LEMON CHICKEN

MAKES 4 SERVINGS

INGREDIENTS

RICE SALAD:

- 2 cups instant brown rice, dry
- 2 cups store-bought organic low-sodium chicken broth
- 1 tablespoon extra-virgin olive oil
- 1 small red onion, diced
- 1 small zucchini, diced
- 1 red bell pepper, diced
- 2 carrots, julienned

- 2 teaspoons lemon juice, freshly squeezed
- Salt (to taste)
- Pepper (to taste)

GRILLED CHICKEN:

- 4 skinless, boneless chicken breast halves
- $\frac{1}{2}$ cup lemon juice, freshly squeezed
- $\frac{1}{2}$ teaspoon salt
- $\frac{1}{4}$ teaspoon pepper
- 2 teaspoons dried parsley

DIRECTIONS

1. Make rice per the instructions, using the chicken broth instead of water; set aside.

2. Heat olive oil in skillet, add all veggies and sauté for 3 minutes.

3. Add rice, and cook on medium heat for 5 minutes. Switch to low heat, and cook until the rice is heated through.

4. Add lemon juice, salt and pepper to taste. Then chill for 30 minutes.

5. While the rice salad is chilling, grill the chicken breasts. Preheat an outdoor grill to medium high, and lightly oil the grate. Dip the chicken in lemon juice, and sprinkle with salt, pepper and parsley.

6. Cook on the prepared grill for 10 to 15 minutes per side or until no longer pink and juices run clear.

7. Serve rice salad cold, and top with freshly sliced grilled chicken. Leftovers can be chilled for the next serving.

Cat Cora

Cat is a chef and lifestyle entrepreneur. She was the first female chef on *Iron Chef America*, which airs on the Food Network. She is the executive chef of *Bon Appétit* and the author of *Cooking from the Hip* and *Cat Cora's Kitchen*.

Cat has a restaurant in Costa Mesa, California, called CCQ, and she has a restaurant at Walt Disney World Resort in Orlando, Florida, called Kouzzina.

Not only is Cat truly talented, but she is also making a difference. After the devastation of the 2004 tsunami in Indonesia, Cat said, "I decided to take on hunger and dedicate energy to connect with others to help bring relief to those in need and provide needed education on nutrition to improve health and well-being." She created Chefs for Humanity and is committed to promoting nutrition education, hunger relief, and emergency and humanitarian aid to reduce hunger worldwide. You can help out, too; visit the Chefs for Humanity website at www.chefsforhumanity.org.

Cat shares six super tantalizing recipes from her book, *Cat Cora's Classics with a Twist*. What I love about Cat's recipes is that they are simple to prepare but look and taste like a cosmopolitan creation.

SMOKED SALMON AND WASABI TEA SANDWICHES

SERVES 6: MAKES 12 SMALL SANDWICHES

Who says tea sandwiches can't be exciting as well as refined? Zingy wasabi, salmon and cream cheese, and cool, crisp cucumber slices give these sandwiches a perfect balance of flavor and color.

I like to use English cucumbers—the long, thin cucumbers that come wrapped in plastic—because they have fewer seeds. I leave on the peel, scrubbing and drying the cuke before slicing it paper-thin, but you can peel it, if you like.

INGREDIENTS

- One 16-ounce brioche loaf (you'll use about half; see note)
- 1 tablespoon wasabi from a tube or $1\frac{1}{2}$ scant teaspoons powdered wasabi
- $\frac{1}{2}$ cup whipped cream cheese (regular or light)
- 4–6 ounces thinly sliced smoked salmon
- 1 large cucumber, preferably English, thinly sliced (see above)
- 1 tablespoon chopped fresh chives

DIRECTIONS

1. Cut twelve 1/2-inch-thick slices of brioche and trim the slices into even squares. Lightly toast the brioche using the lowest setting on your toaster or arrange the bread slices on a baking sheet and toast in an oven set to 350°F for 2 minutes on each side or until lightly colored.

2. In a small bowl, combine the wasabi and cream cheese with a spoon, mixing until the wasabi is completely dispersed. Spread about 1/2 teaspoon of the wasabi cream cheese in a thin, even layer on each slice of bread. Top with a slice of smoked salmon and trim off any excess so the salmon is even with the bread slice all the way around. Top with cucumber slices. Sprinkle with chives. Arrange on a large platter or tray and serve.

Cat's note: If brioche isn't available, try a whole-wheat baguette, party pumpernickel, challah bread, or even slices of sourdough. Because this recipe calls for few ingredients, use good artisan-style bread with a little texture.

Chef's touch: If you're feeling artistic and want a beautifully scalloped top, overlap the cucumber slices on the salmon, like the scales of a fish, and then trim so the sandwiches are even and square.

GRASSHOPPER
MAKES 4 DRINKS

Unlike the saccharine Grasshoppers of the 1960s, my version of this cocktail is lighter and at the same time more complex, thanks to white chocolate liqueur and vanilla-infused vodka. And because I like just a taste of sweet at the end of a meal, sometimes this minty drink is the only dessert I serve. Use clear crème de menthe, which looks better in the glass than the garish green brands.

I use martini glasses, but this cocktail gives you license to be creative and use any glassware you like.

INGREDIENTS

- ½ ounce dark chocolate (60% cocoa or higher)
- 2 teaspoons light corn syrup, for the glass rims
- 6 ounces clear crème de menthe
- 6 ounces white chocolate liqueur (such as Godiva)
- 6 ounces vanilla-infused vodka (such as Absolute)
- 4 small fresh mint sprigs

DIRECTIONS

1. Grate the chocolate, preferably with a microplane grater, onto a saucer. With your finger, run corn syrup around the rim of each glass and roll the rim in the grated chocolate.

2. Pour the crème de menthe, white chocolate liqueur, and vodka into a shaker filled with ice, shake until well-blended, and strain into the glasses, being careful not to splash the chocolate rims. Garnish each cocktail with a sprig of mint.

CURRIED ORANGE LENTIL SOUP   MAKES 4 TO 6 SERVINGS

When I was invited to be on *The Oprah Winfrey Show*, I was asked for a healthy, inexpensive meal, and this soup immediately came to mind. I make it often because it's easy, it's spicy, and you can set out a few garnishing options that make it fun for the kids. I like to add a lot of ginger to this soup, but you can use less or leave it out altogether, if you like.

INGREDIENTS

- 2 tablespoons extra-virgin olive oil
- ½ large onion, chopped
- 2 garlic cloves, chopped
- 2 tablespoons finely chopped fresh ginger (optional)
- 2 teaspoons curry powder
- 1 teaspoon pure chili powder
- ½ teaspoon ground cinnamon
- 1 pound split orange lentils
- 2 cups store-bought low-sodium stock
- 6–8 cups water
- Kosher salt (to taste)
- ½ cup nonfat Greek-style plain yogurt (such as FAGE) or light sour cream
- ½ cup fresh cilantro
- ½ cup chopped scallions
- 1 large lemon, cut into 8 wedges

DIRECTIONS

1. Heat the oil in a large, heavy saucepan set over medium heat. Add the onion and cook slowly, stirring frequently, until golden and soft, about 10 minutes. Add the garlic, ginger, and all the spices and stir well. Cook until the ingredients form a fragrant paste, about 5 minutes. Stir in the lentils. Add the stock and 6 cups of water. Stir well, raise the heat to high, and bring to a boil. Turn the heat to low and cook, stirring occasionally and adding more water if the soup becomes too thick, until the lentils are soft, 40 minutes to 1 hour (check sooner if you used a different variety of lentil).

2. Taste and add salt if necessary. Ladle the soup into bowls, top each serving with a dollop of yogurt or sour cream, and garnish with the cilantro and scallions. Set out the lemon wedges so guests can squeeze in as much juice as they want.

Cat's note: I prefer orange lentils for this soup because they don't taste as earthy as brown lentils, and they're prettier. You can use small French green lentils, if you like, but begin checking after 30 minutes of cooking to see if they are done.

GRILLED AVOCADO COBB SALAD WITH APRICOT DRESSING

MAKES 6 TO 8 SERVINGS

It first occurred to me to grill avocados when I had a bunch of really hard ones that I wanted to use that night. I thought about how to soften them up and, since I grill everything, decided to throw them on and see what happened. I tossed the halves with some olive oil, salt, and pepper, and voilá—avocados with a smoky taste.

For grilling, be sure to choose avocados that are still fairly firm; soft ones don't work.

The apricot preserves are just the right accent for the blue cheese and smoky bacon in the salad.

INGREDIENTS

- 3 large firm avocados, halved, pitted and peeled
- 1 tablespoon extra-virgin olive oil
- Kosher salt and freshly ground black pepper
- 1 1/2 teaspoons fresh lime juice

- 8 cups iceberg, romaine or butter lettuce, chopped
- 1 cup diced tomato
- 1 cup drained, diced, oil-packed sun-dried tomatoes
- 2 large eggs, hard-boiled, peeled, whites and yolks coarsely chopped separately

- 6 slices turkey bacon, cooked and crumbled
- $\frac{1}{2}$ cup crumbled blue cheese

APRICOT DRESSING

- 2 tablespoons white wine vinegar or champagne vinegar

- $\frac{1}{4}$ cup apricot preserves
- $\frac{1}{3}$ cup extra-virgin olive oil
- 1 teaspoon chopped fresh thyme
- Kosher salt and freshly ground black pepper

DIRECTIONS

To grill the avocados: Preheat a gas grill on medium-high heat or light a charcoal grill. Brush or spray the avocados evenly with the olive oil and season them with salt and pepper to taste. Grill the avocado halves just until grill marks form, 2 to 3 minutes. With a spatula, carefully turn the halves and cook for a few minutes more, until marks appear on the other side. Remove to a side dish and sprinkle lime juice over each half. Cool the avocados to room temperature or refrigerate until you're ready to assemble the salad.

For the dressing: In a large bowl, whisk together the vinegar, apricot preserves, olive oil, thyme, and salt and pepper to taste.

To assemble the salad: In a large bowl, toss the lettuce with the dressing. Transfer the dressed lettuce to a large platter. Carefully cut the grilled avocados on the bias into thick slices and place them down the center of the salad. In a small bowl, mix the fresh and sun-dried tomatoes together. Spoon the yolks, whites, bacon, tomatoes, and cheese around the avocado. Serve.

CAT AND MO'S ENCHILADA PIE　　　　MAKES 6 TO 8 SERVINGS

A few years ago, when I started calling myself Cat (short for Cathy), my mom began teasing me by calling herself Mo (short for Mom). Mo is a fantastic cook. This is my take on her enchilada pie. I've given it a dose of fresh cilantro, upped the spices, lowered the fat, and topped it with tortilla chips instead of corn chips. While it bakes, the lowest layers transform into a beefy enchilada-like base, while the top layers stay crisp.

INGREDIENTS

- 1 pound lean ground beef
- 1 medium onion, coarsely chopped

- 2 garlic cloves, minced
- One 10-ounce can enchilada sauce

- One 15-ounce can black beans, drained and rinsed
- Kosher salt (to taste)
- 1 cup light sour cream
- One 4-ounce can chopped green chili peppers, drained
- $\frac{1}{2}$ cup chopped fresh cilantro
- One 12-ounce jar green salsa
- 1 tablespoon pure chili powder

- $1\frac{1}{2}$ teaspoons ground cumin
- 3 cups broken tortilla chips (about the size of corn chips), divided
- 2 cups grated light cheddar, divided
- 3 scallions, chopped (white and light green parts only)
- 2 tablespoons pickled jalapeños, chopped, or 1 tablespoon fresh jalapeños, chopped (optional)
- 2 limes, cut into wedges, for garnish

DIRECTIONS

1. Preheat the oven to 400°F.

2. In a large skillet over medium-high heat, cook the beef, onion, and garlic until the vegetables are soft and the beef is just slightly pink, 6 to 8 minutes. Add the enchilada sauce and black beans, reduce the heat to low and simmer for 10 minutes. Taste and add salt if you like.

3. Meanwhile, in a food processor or blender, blend the sour cream, green chilies, cilantro, salsa, chili powder, and cumin until smooth.

4. Spoon half of the meat-bean mixture into a 9-by-13-inch pan or a large casserole dish. Top with $1\frac{1}{2}$ cups of the smallest of the broken chips and 1 cup of cheese. Cover the chips and cheese with the remaining meat-bean mixture. Spoon on the sour cream mixture and gently spread it to cover the meat in an even layer. Sprinkle on the scallions and the jalapeños, if using. Top with the remaining $1\frac{1}{2}$ cups chips and the remaining 1 cup of cheese. Cover with aluminum foil and bake for 20 minutes. Serve warm, with lime wedges.

NO-BAKE DARK CHOCOLATE GANACHE TARTLETS

MAKES 12 TARTLETS OR 24 MINI TARTLETS

This is the easiest chocolate dessert I know. A touch of cayenne pepper sets off the dark chocolate flavor of the tartlets perfectly, and the no-roll dough for the crust is a snap. This is a great dessert to make the night before you plan to serve it, and if you're going to a party, the tartlets are easy to transport.

The dessert is rich, so I like to make the tartlets in mini-muffin tins, but if all you have is a standard tin, it will work just fine; just cut each tartlet into squares and serve.

If you make the tartlets in very hot weather, decrease the quantity of maple syrup to ½ cup.

INGREDIENTS

CRUST:

- ¾ cup unsweetened cocoa powder
- 1 cup all-purpose flour
- ½ cup maple syrup
- 4 tablespoons (½ stick) unsalted butter, softened
- 1 teaspoon kosher salt

GANACHE FILLING:

- 1 cup unsweetened cocoa powder
- ¾ cup maple syrup (see headnote)
- ½ teaspoon ground cinnamon
- ⅛ – ¼ teaspoon cayenne pepper (optional)
- ½ teaspoon vanilla extract
- 8 tablespoons (1 stick) unsalted butter, melted

DIRECTIONS

1. **For the crust:** Spray a mini-muffin tin or a standard 12-cup muffin tin with nonstick cooking spray.

2. In a stand mixer fitted with a paddle attachment or in a food processor, mix together the cocoa powder, flour, maple syrup, butter, and salt until the mixture begins to hold together and form a dough. Use 2 teaspoons of dough for each mini-muffin cup or 1 heaping tablespoon for each standard-sized cup, flattening the dough into a disk and using your fingers to press the dough onto the bottom and up the sides of each cup. Lightly flour your hands if the dough becomes too sticky. Cover the muffin tin with plastic wrap and refrigerate until well-chilled, at least one hour.

3. **For the filling:** Blend the cocoa powder, maple syrup, cinnamon, cayenne pepper (if using), vanilla, and butter with a whisk in a medium bowl or large measuring cup with a pour spout. Mix until the filling is smooth and no longer grainy. Pour about 2 tablespoons of the filling into the tartlet crust in each of the regular muffin cups or 1 tablespoon into each mini-muffin cup. Refrigerate until completely set, at least 3 hours or preferably overnight.

Twist it: If you like the combination of salt and chocolate, sprinkle a little fleur de sel on the tartlets after they've set. You can also finish each tartlet with a toasted walnut half, a toasted pecan or a sprinkling of cocktail peanuts.

Sheryl Crow

Sheryl is a musician, singer, songwriter and the author of *If It Makes You Healthy* (Macmillan Children's Publishing Group/St. Martin's Press). She has won nine Grammy Awards, performed with the Rolling Stones, and has sung duets with Mick Jagger, Michael Jackson, Eric Clapton, Sting and many others. I personally love her slow-cooked Mojo Criollo Slow-Braised Pork served with rice. Her Vegan Chocolate-Mint Brownies are so tasty it is hard not to eat the entire batch in one sitting—practice portion control. Thank you, Sheryl, for sharing your intoxicating recipes!

MOJO CRIOLLO SLOW-BRAISED PORK   MAKES 6 TO 8 SERVINGS

INGREDIENTS

- 1 cup freshly squeezed lime juice
- 1 cup freshly squeezed orange juice
- 2 tablespoons chopped garlic
- 1 tablespoon dried oregano
- 2 teaspoons kosher salt
- 2 teaspoons freshly ground black pepper
- 1 teaspoon dried red chili flakes

- 1 teaspoon ground cumin
- $\frac{3}{4}$ cup canola oil, preferably expeller-pressed
- 1 bunch scallions, white and green parts, sliced
- $\frac{1}{3}$ cup chopped fresh cilantro leaves
- One 3- to 4-pound boneless Boston butt (pork shoulder), cut into 2 large pieces
- 12 ounces Mexican beer, such as Corona, Dos Equis or Sol

DIRECTIONS

1. In a blender, process the juices, garlic, oregano, salt, pepper, chili flakes and cumin. With the blender on medium speed, slowly drizzle canola oil through the opening in the lid. When the oil is absorbed and the marinade is nicely emulsified, remove the canister from the blender and stir in the scallions and cilantro.

2. Put the pork pieces in a glass, ceramic or other nonreactive dish. Pour the marinade over the pork, cover, and refrigerate for at least 8 hours and up to 12 hours.

3. Preheat the oven to 250°F.

4. Transfer the pork to a disposable aluminum pan. Pour the marinade and the beer over the pork, cover tightly with aluminum foil, and braise until very tender, 6 to 7 hours. The pork is done when it just about falls apart when prodded with a fork. Keep cooking it until it's tender.

5. Shred the pork with 2 forks and your fingers. Serve with rice.

VEGAN CHOCOLATE-MINT BROWNIES   MAKES ABOUT 15 BROWNIES

I like to make Chuck's (chef, coauthor of *If It Makes You Healthy*) vegan brownies at home for Wyatt. I love the fact that they are more healthful than regular brownies and that the hint of mint adds an interesting, fresh taste that both Wyatt and I love. Plus, Wyatt loves licking the spatula!

INGREDIENTS

- 2 cups unbleached all-purpose flour
- 2 cups raw sugar, preferably organic
- $\frac{1}{2}$ cup unsweetened cocoa powder
- 1 teaspoon baking powder
- 1 teaspoon iodized salt

- 1 cup vegetable or canola oil
- 1 to 1 $\frac{1}{2}$ teaspoons peppermint extract
- 1 teaspoon pure vanilla extract
- $\frac{1}{2}$ cup carob chips

DIRECTIONS

1. Preheat the oven to 350°F. Grease a 13-by-9-inch baking pan.

2. In the bowl of an electric mixer fitted with the paddle attachment and set on low speed, mix together the flour, sugar, cocoa powder, baking powder and salt.

3. Once the dry ingredients are mixed together, turn off the motor and add the oil, 1 cup of water, 1 teaspoon of peppermint extract and the vanilla extract. With the mixer on medium-high, beat the batter so that it is well-incorporated and smooth. Taste and add more peppermint extract, if desired. Stir in the carob chips by hand.

4. Pour the batter into the prepared pan and smooth the surface with a rubber spatula. Bake for 25 to 30 minutes or until a toothpick inserted in the center comes out clean.

5. Let the brownies cool in the pan set on a wire rack for 10 to 15 minutes. Cut into squares to serve.

Cristina Ferrare

Cristina is an actress, model, host and the author of *Cristina Ferrare's Big Bowl of Love*. Many may know Cristina as a fashion model who has appeared on the cover of *Vogue, Harper's Bazaar* and *Cosmopolitan*, and she was the face of and spokesperson for Max Factor. I know her as the co-host of the morning show *AM Los Angeles* when I used to model (one of my many careers) when I was in my 20s for their fashion segments, one of which included my cocker spaniel, Scooter, for doggie fashions.

Cristina premiered her new show *Big Bowl of Love* on Oprah Winfrey's network (OWN) on January 3, 2011, with *Eat Like a Woman* contributor and Iron Chef Cat Cora as the show's first guest. *Big Bowl of Love* follows Cristina as she cooks with her friends, family and other guests. She is also featured in a series of cooking videos and blogs on Oprah.com entitled *Cooking with Cristina*.

Her Smashed Yukon Gold Potatoes comfort food recipe has a hint of thyme and truffle salt for a nice finish. They are perfect when served with grilled fish and steamed veggies. For a healthful dessert, treat yourself to Cristina's Phyllo Cups with Greek Yogurt, Fresh Peaches and Honey—they are super tasty.

SMASHED YUKON GOLD POTATOES   MAKES 6 SERVINGS

My grandmother use to make these when I was little, using baby potatoes from the garden. She would cook them in chicken stock, then sauté them in extra-virgin olive oil. I use the Yukon gold or yellow potatoes because I like their buttery texture.

INGREDIENTS

- 12 (about 3-inch by 3-inch) Yukon gold or yellow Dutch potatoes
- 1 quart chicken stock, or store-bought organic chicken broth
- ¼ cup canola oil
- 4 sprigs fresh thyme, one snipped into small pieces
- 1 tablespoon unsalted butter
- Kosher salt (to taste)
- Cracked pepper
- Pinch of truffle salt (optional; you can find truffle salt at specialty grocery stores, or ask your market if they carry it)

DIRECTIONS

1. Place the potatoes in a large saucepan and fill with chicken stock, making sure the stock covers the potatoes by 2 inches. (If you've run out of chicken stock, you can use water.) Bring to a gentle boil and cook for 45 minutes, or until the potatoes are soft enough to run a knife through the center. Drain the potatoes and pat dry.

2. With a wine bottle or olive oil bottle, gently smash the potatoes to flatten them slightly and break open the skins. Heat a skillet (preferably cast iron) for 5 minutes. Add the oil and let heat for 30 seconds. Add the smashed potatoes and fry for about 4 minutes or until the bottoms become crusty. Gently turn over, add sprig of the snipped thyme and fry for 4 minutes. Turn off the heat, add butter, and sprinkle with kosher salt and pepper or truffle salt. Top with remaining thyme leaves and serve immediately.

PHYLLO CUPS WITH GREEK YOGURT, FRESH PEACHES AND HONEY

MAKES 6 SERVINGS

This is a very versatile dessert because you can use any type of fruit you prefer in the recipe. I make mine with Greek yogurt and fresh peaches, but you can substitute your favorite ice cream, frozen yogurt or sorbet.

INGREDIENTS

- Butter-flavored cooking spray
- One 3 ½ ounce package phyllo dough
- ½ cup Greek yogurt
- 3 medium ripe fresh peaches, pitted, skinned and cut into 1-inch pieces
- ¾ teaspoon ground cinnamon
- 2 tablespoons chopped walnuts
- 12 small fresh mint leaves
- 2 tablespoons honey

DIRECTIONS

1. Preheat the oven to 375°F. Spray a 6-cup muffin tin generously with cooking spray.

2. Remove 6 sheets of phyllo from the package, and cover them with a kitchen towel to keep them from drying out. Store the rest of the phyllo dough in the refrigerator.

3. Lay 1 sheet of phyllo dough on a work surface, and keep the remaining sheets covered with a damp towel to prevent them from drying out. Spray the sheet lightly with cooking spray. Cut the sheet into 5 (6-inch by 6-inch) squares. Place 1 square gently inside a muffin cup, and press the bottom to fit into the cup. Lay the other 4 squares in the muffin cup at different angles until all 5 have been gently pressed in. The ends of the phyllo dough will be taller than the cup and should overlap. Repeat the process in the other 5 muffin cups.

4. Bake for 5 to 8 minutes or until golden brown. Remove from the oven and let cool completely before trying to lift the cups from the muffin tins. Gently lift the phyllo cups and place on a platter. Fill each to the top with yogurt. Add half a peach, and sprinkle with ⅛ teaspoon of cinnamon, 1 teaspoon of chopped walnuts, 2 mint leaves torn into small pieces and 1 teaspoon of honey.

Lorena Garcia

Lorena is a chef, restaurateur and the author of *Lorena Garcia's New Latin Classics*. Lorena, who hails from Venezuela, is one of the country's leading Latina chefs. A judge and investor on NBC's *America's Next Great Restaurant* and a guest chef on the season finale of Bravo's *Top Chef All-Stars*, she also competed on season four of Bravo's *Top Chef Masters*. In August 2012, she opened her second traveler's restaurant, Lorena Garcia Tapas, at the Atlanta Airport, in the wake of her flagship Lorena Garcia Cocina in Miami.

Taco Bell recently debuted its new Cantina Bell menu, featuring vibrant flavors and authentic recipes from Garcia's own kitchen.

This busy chef and entrepreneur is also taking on the challenge of childhood obesity with Big Chef, Little Chef, her comprehensive program to help kids and families (visit the website at www.cheflorenagarcia.com/page/big-chef-little-chef). Lorena says, "I was traveling a lot and everywhere I went, I saw an obesity problem, especially in Hispanic families. So I asked myself, 'What can I do to make a difference in kids' lives?'" Today she motivates kids and their parents with healthy food that tastes great.

Lorena creates layers of flavor to create easy-to-make exotic recipes. Her Striped Bass Tacos with Salsa Verde and Corn Peach Salsa will have you drooling for more, and thankfully she shared her Creamy Mango Cups to complete this enticing meal.

STRIPED BASS TACOS WITH SALSA VERDE AND CORN PEACH SALSA — MAKES 6 TO 8 SERVINGS

INGREDIENTS

CITRUS GARLIC STRIPED BASS:

- ¼ cup melted butter
- 1 lemon, juiced, and lemon zest
- 1 tablespoon chili powder
- 4 garlic cloves, finely minced
- ¼ cup chopped fresh cilantro leaves

- 3 tablespoons dill, finely minced
- 1 pound striped bass
- Salt (to taste)
- Pepper (to taste)
- 4-inch corn tortillas

ROASTED SALSA VERDE:

- 3 tomatillos, peeled and cleaned
- 1 jalapeño
- 2 tablespoons olive oil, plus $\frac{1}{4}$ cup for blending
- Salt (to taste)
- Pepper (to taste)
- 1 whole garlic head (roasted)
- 1 bunch cilantro
- 1 lemon, juiced

GRILLED CORN PEACH SALSA:

- 4 charred grilled corn, off the husk after grilling
- 2 small tomatoes, no seeds, small dice
- 2 fresh peaches, small dice
- $\frac{1}{4}$ cup minced red onion
- 2 tablespoons cilantro, chopped
- 2 tablespoons chopped parsley
- 2 cloves garlic, finely minced
- 1 teaspoon fresh lime juice
- 2 teaspoons fresh lemon juice
- 1 teaspoon finely chopped habanero pepper
- Salt (to taste)

DIRECTIONS

1. **For the Citrus Garlic Striped Bass:** In a small saucepan at mid-low heat, add the butter, lemon juice and zest, chili powder, garlic, cilantro and dill, until the butter has melted. Let cool for 5 minutes, place the striped bass on a sheet pan and cover with the butter mixture. Add salt and pepper.

2. Place the fish on a very hot grill or plancha and cook each side for few minutes, until seared and cooked mid well. Set aside until ready to serve; flake the fish with a fork to place on top of a corn tortilla.

3. Warm the tortillas for 20 seconds, add the fish, corn peach salsa and salsa verde (see separate instructions that follow); serve immediately with a lime wedge.

1. **For the Roasted Salsa Verde:** In a mixing bowl, combine tomatillos and jalapeño, and add 2 tablespoons olive oil, salt and pepper.

2. Preheat grill or use side burners of the grill. Add tomatillos and jalapeño, and grill all sides. Cook until tomatillos are soft, about 15 to 20 minutes.

3. Puree the mixture in a blender; add roasted garlic, cilantro, lemon juice and olive oil. Season with salt and pepper to taste.

For the Grilled Corn Peach Salsa: Mix all ingredients together. Serve at room temperature.

CREAMY MANGO CUPS

INGREDIENTS

- 6–7 ripe mangos
- ¾ cup agave syrup, divided
- 1 envelope unflavored gelatin (about 1 tablespoon)
- 1 vanilla bean, halved lengthwise, seeds scraped away and reserved, or 1 teaspoon pure vanilla extract
- 2 tablespoons fresh lemon juice
- 1 cup reduced-fat cream cheese
- Whipped cream (for topping; optional)
- 6 fresh mint sprigs (for serving)

DIRECTIONS

1. Place 5 of the mangos on a cutting board. Using a serrated vegetable peeler or a sharp paring knife, peel, halve, and pit the mangos, then chop them into 1-inch pieces. Place the chopped mangos, ½ cup of the agave syrup, and 1 cup of water in a small saucepan and bring to a simmer over medium-low heat. Cook, stirring occasionally, until the mangos are soft, about 5 minutes. Turn off the heat and set aside.

2. Pour 2 tablespoons of warm water into a small bowl. Sprinkle the gelatin over the water, stir and set aside for 5 minutes to soften.

3. Transfer the mangos and all but 2 tablespoons of the mango juice to a blender jar (set aside the 2 tablespoons mango juice for serving). Add the vanilla bean seeds or the vanilla extract and the gelatin mixture to the blender and process for 1 minute to combine. Add the lemon juice and cream cheese and blend on high speed until the mixture

is silky and smooth, and the texture of the puree is airy and thick, like a mousse, 6 to 8 minutes.

4. Divide the puree among six 4-ounce ramekins and cover each ramekin flush with plastic wrap. Refrigerate until the mixture is set, at least 2 ½ hours or up to 24 hours.

5. Before serving, prepare a medium-low charcoal or gas grill.

6. Halve and pit the remaining mango and place on a large plate. Drizzle the mango with the remaining ¼ cup agave syrup and then grill them cut side down until they have grill marks, about 2 minutes.

7. Remove the ramekins from the refrigerator and top with a dollop of whipped cream, if using. Serve each mango cup on a small plate with a grilled mango on the side. Drizzle the reserved mango juice over the cups. Finish with a mint sprig and serve.

Manouschka Guerrier

Manouschka is a chef, TV personality and the owner of SingleServingBytes.com. A former model, Manouschka learned all she knows about cooking from her mother, Jacqueline, and her Haitian grandmother, Olga, a professionally trained chef. I know her from Food Network's *Private Chefs of Beverly Hills*.

According to her fabulous website SingleServingBytes.com, she has a very impressive list of clients and guests that she has served: Kim Kardashian, Selena Gomez, our very own *Eat Like a Woman* contributor Giuliana Rancic, Barbra Streisand, Donna Karan, James Brolin, and even rocker Meat Loaf.

As the quintessential single, Manouschka owns and operates Los Angeles-based brand Single Serving, where she celebrates the single life and teaches other singles how to serve up chic, easy and affordable meals.

I love her health advice: "Don't skip breakfast. Eat every 3 hours (be it trail mix, blueberries or a protein shake) between meals. Don't eat after 8 p.m. If you need to drink, stay away from dark liquor; stick to vodka soda with a lime." Manouschka loves a good Philly cheesesteak, cheeseburgers, potato chips and bacon—this is one honest lady!

She is committed to Partners in Health of Haiti, where they operate clinics and hospitals to provide options for the poor. The executive director and cofounder says, "We believe that love and imagination are potent weapons in the fight for the poor." Find out more on the website at www.pih.org/country/haiti.

Manouschka shares a typical menu in her day with the recipe for Avocado Toast. She demonstrates that it is easy to eat like a woman. This recipe kept me feeling full for hours. Ezekiel bread is so good for you—it contains no flour, is a wonderful source of protein and fiber and is great for keeping your blood sugar stable. Avocados, flaxseeds and extra-virgin olive oil—this breakfast is packed with great ingredients and is so easy to make.

For lunch, Manouschka suggested quinoa salad with cranberries and kale with a citrus vinaigrette. For a snack, she likes the trail mix from Whole Foods. And for dinner, she'd opt for a roasted turkey leg and a watercress salad, along with a glass (or three) of Malbec (a yummy mid-bodied red wine originally from France but now grown in Argentina and Chile). And for dessert? A spoonful of Trader Joe's Cookie Butter.

AVOCADO TOAST

MAKES 1 SERVING

INGREDIENTS

- ½ avocado, mashed with a fork
- ½ lime, juiced
- 1 teaspoon ground flaxseed
- ¼ teaspoon red pepper flakes
- Sea salt (to taste)
- Cracked pepper (to taste)
- 2 slices Ezekiel bread (toasted)
- Extra-virgin olive oil (to taste)

DIRECTIONS

In a bowl, mash avocado; add lime juice, flaxseed, red pepper flakes. Season with course sea salt and fresh cracked pepper; spread on toast. Drizzle with extra-virgin olive oil.

Florence Henderson

Florence is an actress, singer and the author of *Florence Henderson's Short-Cut Cooking*. We all know her as America's favorite Mom—Carol Brady on the ABC sitcom *The Brady Bunch*—and recently a contestant on *Dancing with the Stars*. Today she has her own talk show, *The Florence Henderson Show* on RLTV.

I had the good fortune of meeting Florence when I post-produced a Lifetime TV program, "Speaking of Women's Health." Florence was the host, with Rachel Campos.

Florence's guilty food pleasure is, "Pasta, pasta, pasta." Her advice for all is, "Keep a cool head and a warm heart." I have personally witnessed that she walks her talk.

Her favorite causes are the City of Hope cancer research hospital and the House Research Institute. You can find out more about Florence on her website at FloHome.com.

You will love her easy-to-follow recipes. They are wholesome and healthy—maybe that is her secret to keeping that girlish figure.

SATURDAY LUNCH
WALDORF CHICKEN SALAD

MAKES 4 TO 6 SERVINGS

This traditional salad lends itself to any number of variations according to what you have in your pantry: golden raisins, dried cherries or currants, jicama, pears, carrots, or onions would all be delicious. I think this dish makes a lovely no-fuss weekend lunch for family or guests. Again, experiment and enjoy!

INGREDIENTS

- 3 cups chopped, cooked chicken meat
- $\frac{1}{2}$ cup chopped celery
- $\frac{1}{2}$ cup chopped apples (use whatever variety is in season in your supermarket)
- $\frac{1}{2}$ cup seedless red or green grape halves
- $\frac{1}{2}$ cup chopped salt-free cashews (or use pecans or walnuts)

- Juice of 1 lemon
- $\frac{1}{4}$ cup sour cream (or fat-free yogurt)
- $\frac{1}{2}$ cup regular or low-fat mayonnaise
- 1 tablespoon chopped fresh dill
- Salt (to taste)
- Freshly ground black pepper (to taste)
- Bibb lettuce leaves

DIRECTIONS

1. Place the chicken meat in a mixing bowl.

2. Add the celery, apples, grape halves and nuts. Toss together lightly.

3. Drizzle the lemon juice over the mixture.

4. Add the sour cream and mayonnaise and toss well. (Add a bit more of each if you like a salad mixture with more moisture.) Add the fresh dill and stir to combine. Add the salt and pepper to taste.

5. To serve, place the lettuce leaves on plates and top each serving with a mound of the chicken salad. Serve immediately or cover and chill for an hour before serving. Add a loaf of crusty bread and some wine for a fabulous lunch.

ZESTY HOT NUTS
THIS RECIPE HAS NO SET AMOUNTS—
JUST USE WHAT LOOKS RIGHT FOR THE NUMBER OF GUESTS YOU EXPECT.

Like most people who travel frequently by airplane, I've sampled many a snack of mixed nuts. Most people seem to love them as much as I do, so I thought I'd serve a spiced-up version of them at home, too. My sister Ilean and her husband, Ed, send us a huge tin of mixed nuts every year, which Ed hulls himself, and the almonds are my favorite. Putting together this appetizer couldn't be simpler if you buy the ingredients in packages. These are great with cocktails, especially margaritas, which are another specialty of mine—according to my guests!

INGREDIENTS

- Pesto sauce (premade from the supermarket)
- Whole almonds
- Whole cashews
- Whole peanuts
- Pecan halves
- Walnut halves
- Any other nuts you like: hazelnuts, macadamia nuts, etc.
- Ground cayenne pepper

DIRECTIONS

1. In a nonstick skillet over medium-high heat, add enough pesto sauce to coat all of the nuts and stir.

2. Add the nuts to the pesto sauce, and toss in the skillet until all the nuts are thoroughly coated, about 1 minute.

3. Remove the skillet from the heat and sprinkle the cayenne pepper to taste over the nuts. Cool the nuts on paper towels spread out on a flat surface. Serve in small bowls, strategically located throughout your entertaining areas.

SIMPLE SUNDAY SUPPER POT ROAST

MAKES 6 SERVINGS (OR 2 SERVINGS WITH LOTS OF LEFTOVERS TO WORK WITH)

My dad made the best pot roast, and I think he'd be pleased with his daughter's easy-to-prepare recipe. It just pops in the oven to cook with no fuss and no muss. I call it a "smart supper," since the leftovers can last into the following week. Roast beef sandwiches, vegetable beef soup, and roast beef hash are just a few of the great, quick meals that can be made with the leftovers. Thanks, Dad, for starting a great tradition!

INGREDIENTS

- One 4-pound chuck or bottom round roast (or rump or brisket), rinsed and patted dry
- 3 cloves garlic, crushed
- ½ cup flour seasoned with salt, black pepper, paprika and chopped fresh parsley
- 3 tablespoons good-quality olive oil
- 1 bag baby carrots (about 24 carrots)
- 4 Yukon Gold potatoes, unpeeled, quartered
- 1 bunch scallions, trimmed and cut into 4 sections
- 2 ribs celery, chopped
- 1 cup beef or vegetable broth
- 1 cup white wine (or substitute nonalcoholic wine or additional broth)
- 2 bay leaves

DIRECTIONS

1. Preheat the oven to 350°F.

2. Rub the outside of the roast with the crushed garlic. Shake the seasoned flour over the roast, turning to coat it all well.

3. In a large roasting pan over medium-high heat on top of the stove, heat the olive oil.

4. Add the roast to the roasting pan and cook, turning on all sides, until it is golden brown. Remove the pan from the stove and turn the heat off.

5. Scatter the carrots, potatoes, scallions and celery around and over the roast in the pan.

6. Pour the broth and wine around the roast and add the bay leaves.

7. Cover the roasting pan with a lid, or aluminum foil, and bake in the oven for $1\frac{1}{2}$ to 2 hours. Cut into the meat to check doneness. Remove the cover and bake for another 30 minutes.

8. Remove the bay leaves and serve slices or chunks of the roast with vegetables and pot juices. It's wonderful served with some crusty bread to mop up the juices.

FREE-FORM APPLE-BERRY TART

MAKES 8 SERVINGS

Since I have fond memories of picking berries as a kid, I always find fruit tarts to be a satisfying way to finish a meal. If you want this tart to be ready for you at the end of yours, assemble it at the same time that you prepare the rest of your food, and then pop it in the oven about midway through eating. You'll be ready for each other right on time! If you don't have blueberries or raspberries, use any fruit or berries you enjoy to make free-form tarts—pears, apricots, peaches, raspberries, strawberries or blackberries. They're all delicious!

INGREDIENTS

- 1 premade piecrust (from the refrigerator section of the supermarket)
- 1 pound apples (Gala, Rome, Granny Smith, or Braeburn are all wonderful)
- $\frac{1}{2}$ pint fresh or whole frozen blueberries
- $\frac{1}{2}$ pint fresh or whole frozen raspberries
- 2 tablespoons lemon juice

- 3 tablespoons granulated sugar, divided
- 1 teaspoon ground cinnamon
- 2 tablespoons all-purpose flour
- 1 tablespoon unsalted butter, chilled and cut into very small pieces
- Powdered sugar to sprinkle on top of cooked tart

DIRECTIONS

1. On a lightly floured surface, roll the piecrust dough out into a rough circle, about 14 inches in diameter. Place the dough circle on a baking sheet, cover with plastic wrap and chill while you prepare the filling.

2. Core the apples and cut them into $\frac{1}{4}$-inch slices. You'll need about 2 cups of fruit. Place the slices in a glass mixing bowl.

3. Add the blueberries, raspberries and lemon juice and toss gently.

4. Sprinkle 2 tablespoons of the sugar and the cinnamon over all and toss gently.

5. In a separate small bowl, mix together the remaining tablespoon of sugar and the flour. Set the mixture aside.

6. Preheat the oven to 400°F.

7. Remove the chilled piecrust from the refrigerator, take off the plastic wrap, and sprinkle the crust with the sugar-flour mixture. Leave a 2-inch border all around.

8. Arrange the fruit mixture evenly over the sugar-flour mixture, still leaving a 2-inch border. Fold the sides of the crust over the fruit, overlapping where necessary. Brush to folded areas of the crust with water and press them together. This creates the sides of the tart. The center area of the tart will be open. Scatter the butter pieces over the filling.

9. Bake the tart in the oven for about 30 minutes. Cover the outer edge of the crust with foil if it begins to get brown too quickly. The tart should be golden brown and bubbly, with the apples softened. Remove the tart from the oven and let it cool for about 10 minutes before servings.

When cooled down a bit, sift some powdered sugar over all. Cut the tart into wedges and serve.

Linda Hogan

Linda is an actress, television personality, entrepreneur, owner of Sunny Girl Avocados, an animal rights activist and the author of *Wrestling the Hulk: My Life Against the Ropes*.

Linda starred on the hit reality TV show *Hogan Knows Best*. Because of her on- and off-screen devotion to her family, she quickly became one of America's favorite moms.

After a widely publicized divorce, Linda found the strength to rebuild her life and not look back. She encourages women everywhere that they can live and love again at any age.

An animal lover and activist, Linda teamed up with People for the Ethical Treatment of Animals (PETA) in 2010 to protest against animal abuse in the circus. She continues to be involved with this important cause as well as the American Society for the Prevention of Cruelty to Animals (online at www.aspca.org).

Linda divides her time between Miami and Los Angeles and is busy launching an upcoming skin care and clothing line, as well as owning and operating her own farm, Sunny Girl Avocados in Southern California.

I have never met a person who owned an avocado farm, but it explains why her recipes, Three Amigos Guacamole and Grape Salsa, are out of this world. She includes great tips, and I plan on practicing them all, including having a friend make you a margarita.

Avocados promote heart health and have anti-inflammatory benefits—enjoy.

You can learn more about Linda at www.LindaHogan.com.

THREE AMIGOS GUACAMOLE   MAKES 3 TO 4 SERVINGS

INGREDIENTS

- ½ cup chopped yellow onion
- 4 Serrano chilies
- ¼ cup chopped cilantro
- ¾ cup tomato (no seeds or juice), well drained
- 2 teaspoons salt
- ¼ cup lime juice, or squeeze two fresh limes
- 4 large, ripe, fresh California Haas avocados, hopefully hand-picked from my farm! (cut avocados in half, remove the seeds, but save the seeds for later!)
- 3 friends

DIRECTIONS

1. In a food processor, combine onion, chilies, cilantro, tomatoes, salt and lime juice. Puree, then pour into a mixing bowl.

2. Scoop out avocados with a tablespoon, and fold into the mixture.

3. Now sit down. Have one friend clean up, one friend make you a margarita and the other friend serve the food. *Then,* let everyone eat!!

4. Serve guacamole with corn tortilla chips. (I love Tostitos Hint of Lime, and my favorite grape salsa!)

5. Add the avocado seeds to your finished bowl of guacamole and leave them in—I swear the guacamole will *not* turn brown, even overnight!!

GRAPE SALSA

MAKES 1 TO 2 SERVINGS

The spicy-hot chili and crunchy onion, blended with the cool cilantro and sweet grapes, is absolutely delicious and so addictive, you *will* eat the whole bowl of salsa and the entire bag of chips yourself!!

INGREDIENTS

- 1 cup cold seedless red and green grapes (rinsed and separated from stem)
- 1 jalapeño
- ½ red onion
- 1 cup cilantro
- 2 teaspoons salt
- 1 teaspoon lemon juice

DIRECTIONS

Blend all of the ingredients in a food processor and puree; then pour into a serving bowl and serve with corn tortilla chips!

Padma Lakshmi

Padma is an actress, model, host and the author of *Tangy Tart Hot & Sweet*. She has been a host of the Emmy Award–winning reality-competition series *Top Chef* since 2006. She was born in India but grew up in the United States. After a modeling agent discovered her in Spain, Padma modeled for famous designers such as Armani, Versace and Ralph Lauren, and she says, "I was the first Indian model to have a career in Paris, Milan and New York."

Modeling led to acting jobs, including a part in the Italian miniseries, *Caraibi*, which required her to gain 30 pounds. After the job, she lost the weight and published a cookbook, *Easy Exotic*, with recipes incorporating the flavors of Southeast Asia. The book was so successful that the Food Network produced her show, *Padma's Passport*.

She also has her own line of Indian-inspired jewelry, and a line of spices and bakeware. Her newest project is daughter, Krishna. Padma is one busy lady who creates imaginative recipes that are so good for you.

TUNA AND RED BEAN SALAD
MAKES 4 TO 6 SERVINGS

This is one of those versatile salads that makes a great lunch for 4, served with just some freshly baked bread, or a nice, light starter for 6 people. It's great for summer because the only cooking involves lighting the grill. It's also healthy enough to help you prepare for bathing suit season.

INGREDIENTS

DRESSING:

- Juice of 1 very ripe lemon
- $\frac{1}{4}$ cup olive oil
- 2 teaspoons balsamic vinegar
- $\frac{1}{2}$ teaspoon dried oregano
- Salt (to taste)

TUNA:

- 12-ounce tuna steak, about 1-inch thick
- 5 ounces mixed baby lettuces and field greens

- 10 ounces fresh or frozen artichoke bottoms, blanched if frozen; scraped and cored, steamed, and quartered if fresh
- 1 cup sliced English cucumber
- 1 cup halved cherry or grape tomatoes
- $\frac{1}{2}$ cup fresh-snipped chives
- $\frac{1}{2}$ cup chopped fresh flat-leaf parsley
- One 10-ounce can red kidney beans, drained and rinsed

DIRECTIONS

1. Light the grill so that the coals get nice and hot. When the flames have died down and the coals are glowing red and white, sear the tuna on the grill for about 3 minutes on each side; the exact time will depend on the tuna's thickness and how rare you want it.

2. Mix all the dressing ingredients in a small bowl or screw-top jar.

3. Lay a bed of lettuce and field greens in a large salad bowl or platter.

4. In a separate bowl, toss together the artichokes, cucumbers, tomatoes, chives, parsley and kidney beans.

5. Spoon this vegetable mixture in a mound in the center of the greens.

6. Slice the tuna steak into $\frac{1}{4}$-inch slices. Lay the slices decoratively over the mound of vegetables.

   Just before serving, drizzle the dressing evenly over the salad.

Reprinted with permission from Weinstein Books.

TEA SANDWICHES WITH GOAT CHEESE AND CUCUMBER

MAKES 4 TO 6 SERVINGS

Okay, so most of us don't sit around and have afternoon tea anymore, but these graceful little triangles dotted with garnet jewels of pomegranate and grassy notes of cucumber and dill demand an occasion worthy of them. They can be made so easily and are perfect for whipping up whenever guests descend unexpectedly. I agree most of us don't keep shelled pomegranates in our fridge, but many of the better grocery stores often sell pre-peeled pomegranate seeds near the sliced melon in the produce section. Pomegranates are mostly available in the fall; you can substitute dried cranberries or cherries for them the rest of the year. If the dried berries are large, chop them up into morsels first. The taste is different but just as scrumptious.

INGREDIENTS

- 10 thin, square slices of good white bread, grilled or toasted on both sides
- $\frac{1}{4}$ teaspoon olive oil
- 2 ounces goat cheese, about a 2-inch cube
- 2 to 3 teaspoons dill
- Fresh pomegranate seeds
- 40 $\frac{1}{8}$-inch-thick slices of English cucumber, approximately half the cucumber

DIRECTIONS

1. Place the toast on a platter.

2. Combine the olive oil, goat cheese and dill. Spread this paste evenly onto the toast.

3. Sprinkle with the pomegranate seeds, gently pressing them into the cheese.

4. Place 4 slices of cucumber on top of the cheese on each slice of toast.

5. Carefully cut each slice diagonally to make triangles. Ideally two of the four cucumber slices will also be cut in half. These are best served open-faced and arranged on a platter. They're great with afternoon tea or to accompany cocktails.

Reprinted with permission from Weinstein Books.

TWO HENS LAUGHING

MAKES 4 SERVINGS

The delicate flavor of Cornish game hens makes this a one-of-a-kind dish that is just right for a special occasion. I used to make it for family gatherings where we would all sit around thinking up names Confucius may have used to describe things. This one stuck.

INGREDIENTS

- 2 tablespoons canola oil
- 1 teaspoon black mustard seeds
- 1 teaspoon fenugreek seeds
- 1 teaspoon crushed red pepper
- $\frac{1}{2}$ teaspoon asafetida powder
- 1 navel orange cut into 8 pieces, peeled and seeded
- $\frac{1}{4}$ cup fresh kumquats, halved and seeded
- 3 cups 1-inch cubes of day-old bread with crusts
- $\frac{1}{4}$ cup coarse sea or rock salt

- 1 tablespoon anar dana (dried pomegranate seeds; optional)
- 1 tablespoon finely grated orange peel
- 2 tablespoons honey
- 2 tablespoons chopped fresh dill
- 1 tablespoon toasted sesame oil
- 1 teaspoon cayenne
- $\frac{1}{2}$ teaspoon sambar curry powder (or Madras curry powder)
- 2 Cornish game hens, innards removed

DIRECTIONS

1. Preheat the oven to 350°F.

2. In a small wok, heat the canola oil over medium-high heat. Add the mustard seeds. When they start to pop and crackle, add the fenugreek seeds, crushed red pepper and asafetida powder. After 2 to 3 minutes, add orange and kumquats; stir. Cook for 4 to 5 minutes, stirring.

3. Add cubed bread and just enough salt to taste. Stir-fry the bread and citrus mixture for 4 to 7 more minutes, just until the flavors mix well into

a doughy mass. Remove from the heat and stir in the anar dana, if you are using it. Set aside.

4. Place the orange peel, honey, chopped dill, sesame oil, cayenne and sambar powder in a bowl; stir together vigorously to form a paste. Set aside.

5. Wash the hens, and pat them very dry with paper towels.

6. Rub the skins of the hens very well with sea salt.

7. Stuff the cavity of the hens with the bread mixture and place them in a baking dish. Cook the hens in the preheated oven. After 7 minutes, turn the pan around for even cooking. After 5 more minutes, remove and glaze hens well with the orange peel paste. Bake for an additional 15 to 20 minutes, basting often. Uncover for the last 5 to 7 minutes to roast the skins well.

8. Scoop out the stuffing; if necessary to cook out any excess moisture, place it in another baking pan and return it to the oven for a few additional minutes. Meanwhile, place the hens facing each other on a large platter, with the legs facing the edge of the platter.

9. Spoon the stuffing around the birds. Serve hot, and carve tableside.

Reprinted with permission from Weinstein Books.

PEACHES IN RED WINE
MAKES 6 SERVINGS

This is a great recipe to whip up on the spur of the moment in summer during peach season. There are many variations of this jewel of a dish, all worth gobbling up. For instance, in the winter, you could use pears and white wine or Moscato dessert wine with cloves. If you have trouble finding the Recioto, which is an Italian dessert wine from Valpolicella, use a dry red wine of your choice and add a sprinkle of sugar, if needed. Port is also an excellent stand-in.

INGREDIENTS

- 3 cinnamon sticks
- 5 ripe peaches, peeled, pitted and quartered
- $1\frac{1}{2}$ cups Recioto red dessert wine or port

DIRECTIONS

Lay the cinnamon sticks at the bottom of a bowl and place the peaches on top. Pour in the wine, making sure it covers all of the fruit. Marinate in the fridge for at least 2 hours. Serve in small dessert bowls.

Reprinted with permission from Weinstein Books.

Lisa Lillien

Lisa is the creator of the Hungry Girl brand, founder of Hungry-Girl.com, a best-selling author, a producer and a TV host. I have been a fan of Lisa, a.k.a. Hungry Girl, since the beginning. Her claim is that she is not a nutritionist—she is just hungry—but this girl knows food! She even calls herself a "foodologist." Lisa writes a weekly column on WeightWatchers.com, contributes to *Redbook* magazine, and appears on all the TV talk shows, including *The Dr. Oz Show.*

Lisa takes ingredients we love and creates healthy low-calorie recipes so you can enjoy them guilt-free. Today she has her own TV show, *Hungry Girl,* that airs on both the Food Network and Cooking Channel. A million subscribers and I love her daily email with new recipes, tips and tricks.

In all her success, Lisa has always responded to my personal emails. She even gave me advice on how to be calm before my appearance on *The Today Show* for my first book. I am so happy she has shared a couple of her super-delicious recipes that sneak out a few calories while keeping them yummy.

Lisa's guilty food pleasures are pizza and French fries, but she quickly adds, "but not together!" Her health advice is, "walk as much as you can…take the stairs!" She is a big supporter of animal charities and rescues.

If you ever have a chance to attend one of her book signings, I promise it will be the most fun event you have attended at a bookstore. Lisa is the master of "real-food eating situations."

Check out her website at Hungry-Girl.com.

APPLE CRISP IN A MUG   MAKES 1 SERVING

INGREDIENTS

- 1 tablespoon old-fashioned oats
- $\frac{1}{2}$ teaspoon light whipped butter or light buttery spread
- 1 dash nutmeg
- 1 dash salt

- 1 tablespoon brown sugar (not packed), divided
- 1 tablespoon whole-wheat flour, divided
- $\frac{1}{4}$ teaspoon plus 1 dash cinnamon
- $1\frac{1}{2}$ cups peeled and chopped Fuji apples
- Optional topping: fat-free Reddi-wip

DIRECTIONS

1. In a small microwave-safe bowl, combine oats, butter, nutmeg and salt. Add 2 teaspoons brown sugar, 1 teaspoon flour and a dash of cinnamon. Mash and stir until well-mixed and crumbly. Microwave for 30 seconds or until firm.

2. Place apples in a large microwave-safe mug sprayed with nonstick spray. Sprinkle with remaining 1 teaspoon brown sugar, 2 teaspoons flour and 1/4 teaspoon cinnamon. Stir to coat. Microwave for 4 minutes or until apples are tender.

3. Stir oat mixture, breaking it into pieces, and sprinkle over the apple mixture. Mmmm!

From *Hungry Girl 200 under 200 Just Desserts: 200 Recipes Under 200 Calories.*

COOL 'N' CRUNCHY SALMON TACOS   MAKES 1 SERVING

INGREDIENTS

* 2 tablespoons fat-free sour cream
* 1 teaspoon ranch dressing/dip seasoning mix
* One 2.6-ounce pouch boneless, skinless pink salmon, roughly flaked (about 1/2 cup)
* 2 tablespoons finely chopped onion
* 1/4 cup peeled and finely chopped cucumber
* 1/2 tablespoon chopped fresh dill
* 2 corn tacos
* 1/4 cup shredded lettuce
* 1/4 cup diced tomato

DIRECTIONS

1. In a medium bowl, thoroughly mix sour cream with ranch seasoning. Add salmon, onion, cucumber and dill, and stir to coat.

2. Divide salmon mixture between taco shells. Top with lettuce and tomato and eat!

Taco Shell Tip: Look for flat-bottomed shells. They're easier to work with.

From *Hungry Girl to the Max!: The Ultimate Guilt-Free Cookbook.*

Dolly Parton

Dolly is a singer-songwriter, actress, philanthropist and author of *Dolly's Dixie Fixin's*. I am so excited to share a recipe from Dolly Parton—yes, you read that right, *the* Dolly Parton. Her Hello Dolly Bars are a perfect sweet treat during your *Eat Like a Woman* day.

I have been a fan my entire life; Dolly has been such an inspiration. She began her grassroots country career at the age 12 and went on to be a great country music superstar and prolific songwriter.

"Jolene" is still one of my favorite songs, inspired by a tall, redheaded bank teller who Parton believed was flirting with her husband, and her husband's apparent vulnerability to the teller's charm as indicated by his sudden interest in making frequent trips to the bank. She won a Grammy Award for Best Female Country Vocal Performance for her "Here You Come Again."

Dolly went on to star in movies, including *9 to 5*, *The Best Little Whorehouse in Texas*, *Rhinestone* and, my favorite, *Steel Magnolias*. From the Grand Ole Opry to Hollywood, she made it big.

It wasn't until my husband, Michael Becker, was Oscar nominated for best song in a movie, *Crash*, that I finally got within three rows of her. She was also nominated for the same category—how crazy is that? Michael said, "If I lose, it's okay to lose to Dolly."

When I invited Dolly to submit a recipe, I got a glimpse into her passion—reading. The Dollywood Foundation and the Imagination Library (http://usa.imaginationlibrary.com) both promote the love for reading in young children. She has been honored as a living legend by the Library of Congress, and continues to sell out concerts around the world.

She embraces good old-fashioned food and these Hello Dolly Bars will knock your socks off. You will need to practice portion control, or increase your time at the gym—but these bars are worth it.

HELLO DOLLY BARS   MAKES A DOZEN BARS

These are fun to make because there's little more to them than puttin' the ingredients in a pan and baking them up. Don't worry if they look soggy when they come out of the oven; they firm up as they cool.

INGREDIENTS

- 8 tablespoons (1 stick) butter, melted
- 1 cup graham cracker crumbs
- 1 cup chocolate chips
- 1 cup sweetened shredded coconut
- 1 cup chopped pecans
- One 14-ounce can sweetened condensed milk

DIRECTIONS

1. Preheat the oven to 350°F.

2. Pour the butter into an 8-by-8-inch baking pan. Spread the graham cracker crumbs in the bottom of the pan. Arrange the chocolate chips over the crumbs, followed by the coconut and pecans.

3. Bake until golden, about 20 minutes. The bars will not look like they're cooked; they need to cool on a rack to firm up. Cut into bars once cooled.

Giuliana Rancic

Giuliana is an E! news anchor, *Fashion Police* cohost, costar of reality TV series *Giuliana and Bill* (with her husband Bill Rancic, an *Apprentice* winner), author of *Think Like a Guy* and *I Do, Now What?*, and entertainment journalist.

I know Giuliana as the coanchor of *E! News* with Ryan Seacreast. She has also appeared on the red carpet for the Oscars, Grammys and Golden Globes, interviewing stars and getting the scoop on fashion, diet, fitness and even travel tips.

In 2011, Giuliana was diagnosed with early-stage breast cancer, and ultimately decided to have a double mastectomy. Loved by many, including her 3 million Twitter followers, Giuliana is committed to health and recently launched her health and wellness newsletter, *FitFabFun*.

Giuliana has partnered with Bright Pink, a nonprofit organization that focuses on the risk reduction and early detection of breast and ovarian cancer in young women, and provides support for high-risk individuals (find out more online at www.brightpink.org/ive-been-diagnosed/fab-u-wish).

Giuliana's Tuscan Kale and Heirloom Spinach Salad can be enjoyed for lunch, dinner or even as a snack. The ingredients are vitamin-rich, and it is easy to make.

You can learn more about Giuliana at www.GiulianaRancic.com.

TUSCAN KALE AND HEIRLOOM SPINACH SALAD

MAKES 2 SERVINGS

INGREDIENTS

SALAD:

- 1 cup Tuscan kale, hand torn into bite-sized pieces
- 2 cups heirloom spinach, hand torn into bite-sized pieces
- 1 tablespoon cherry peppers, stems and seeds removed, small dice
- 1 tablespoon French breakfast radishes, washed, thinly sliced
- 1 tablespoon celery leaves
- $\frac{1}{4}$ cup Pecorino cheese, grated
- $\frac{1}{4}$ cup lemon-mustard vinaigrette (recipe follows)

- $\frac{1}{4}$ teaspoon lemon zest
- Salt (to taste)
- Pepper (to taste)

VINAIGRETTE:

- 2 tablespoons Dijon mustard
- $\frac{1}{4}$ cup lemon juice
- $\frac{3}{4}$ cup salad oil
- $\frac{1}{4}$ cup extra-virgin olive oil
- Salt (to taste)
- Pepper (to taste)

DIRECTIONS

1. Place kale, spinach, cherry peppers, radishes, celery leaves, cheese and vinaigrette in a mixing bowl. Carefully mix together. Season with salt.

2. Whisk together the vinaigrette ingredients until emulsified. Season with salt and pepper.

3. Mound the salad on a serving plate, dress with the vinaigrette, grate lemon over the top and season with freshly cracked black pepper.

Delilah Winder

Delilah is a celebrity chef, entrepreneur and author of *Delilah's Everyday Soul: Southern Cooking with Style*. Delilah has been Southern cooking with style all her life, but the world got to witness her gift when Oprah Winfrey announced her macaroni and cheese dish as the "best of the best" dish in the country. (No, that recipe is not *Eat Like a Woman*-approved, but it sure sounds tempting!)

Delilah says, "I need to cook in the same way a painter needs to paint or a writer needs to write…cooking and eating are soulful endeavors." Her favorite guilty food pleasure is "hot, crisp French fries with hot sauce, not pepper sauce."

Delilah has served as a celebrity judge for events supporting the Coalition Against Hunger, an organization to fight hunger and promote nutrition (visit the website at www.hungercoalition.org).

In 2000, she opened the elegant Bluezette restaurant that embraces her Southern heritage. Later, she launched two other restaurants, Delilah's Southern Cuisine in her hometown, Philadelphia.

Delilah has been a favorite chef to celebrities such as Patti LaBelle, Denzel Washington, Danny Glover and Tavis Smiley. She has appeared on *The Oprah Winfrey Show*, the Food Network and NBC's *Today Show*.

Delilah shares a summer menu created to nourish your body and soul. Steamed Blue Crabs with Grilled Corn on the Cob and Baked Beans are followed by refreshing Pineapple Sherbet.

STEAMED BLUE CRABS   MAKES 4 SERVINGS

Almost everyone loves crab, but as far as whole steamed crabs go, either you don't touch 'em or you love 'em. People who can't be bothered with steamed crabs (you know who you are!) complain that they require just too much time and energy for so little reward. They want the crab, but they don't want to do the work. Folks who love whole crabs, however, are crazy, not only about the flavor of the incomparably sweet meat, but the whole eating routine as well. They'll sit for hours with a pile of crabs, cracking, picking and sucking away at the shells for the teeniest drop of juice or most miniscule piece of meat. In addition to this admirable patience, the truest connoisseurs also have all kinds of serious rituals. Some only like male crabs (jimmies), while others prefer females (sooks). Some pick all the claws off, pile them up, and eat them first. Others do the same with the bodies. Still other folks painstakingly suck all of the meat and juice out of the tediously tender legs, while some just throw them out. The variety of routines is as great as the number of hours these people can sit in one place.

Most of the crabs we eat in the mid-Atlantic region come from the Chesapeake Bay area and are available throughout the summer. In my opinion, the meatiest and most flavorful crabs are caught from late August to early September. Outside of the summer season, most crabs are likely coming from Louisiana, where they are heavy and full of meat most of the year.

I do hope you have some steamed crab lovers in your midst. This really is a fun and easy recipe, and nothing says summer like cracking open a pile of crabs with some ice-cold beer and good friends.

INGREDIENTS

- Two 12-ounce bottles beer
- $\frac{1}{2}$ cup apple cider vinegar
- 4 cups water

- 24 live Maryland blue crabs, preferably large jimmies
- 2 cups Old Bay seasoning, divided
- 3 dried bay leaves

DIRECTIONS

1. Pour the beer, vinegar and water into a large stockpot. Add half of the crabs, sprinkle with 1 cup of Old Bay, and place the bay leaves on top. Arrange the rest of the crabs over the seasonings and sprinkle with the remaining 1 cup of Old Bay. Cover and bring to a boil over medium-high heat. Reduce the heat to medium and simmer until the crabs are bright red, about 14 to 16 minutes.

2. Set a large colander in a large bowl and drain the crabs, reserving the steaming liquid.

3. To serve, arrange the crabs on a large serving platter and pour the steaming liquid into small bowls for dipping.

GRILLED CORN ON THE COB   MAKES 6 SERVINGS

No wonder summer is my favorite time of year—it is the season for corn, and I am crazy about corn. For purists like myself, eating it hot off the cob is the best. There is just nothing like biting into an ear of perfectly cooked corn, the kernels cracking between your teeth and bursting with sweet juice in every bite. What is better than that?

Boiled or steamed corn is fine, but I think grilling it is even better. By grilling the ears in the husks (with the silk removed), the kernels become just tender and develop a roasted flavor, while remaining protected from the high heat. As I suggest in this recipe, I like brushing the ears with a little butter and seasoning them with some salt and pepper, but that's it. There is no need to get fancy here. If the corn is fresh and sweet, it surely doesn't require anything else. Once you've had grilled corn, you might never want to cook it on the stove again.

INGREDIENTS

- 6 ears fresh corn, husks on
- 12 tablespoons (1 $\frac{1}{2}$ sticks) butter
- Salt (to taste)
- Black pepper (to taste)

DIRECTIONS

1. Prepare a hot grill.

2. Carefully husk the corn, keeping the husks attached at the stems and removing the silk. Rub each ear of corn with 2 tablespoons of butter, pull the husks back up around the buttered corn, and place on the grill. Turn the ears every 2 to 3

minutes until well-browned, about 10 to 15 minutes total.

To serve, pull back the husks from the hot corn, season with salt and pepper, and pile on a serving platter.

BAKED BEANS   MAKES 10 SERVINGS

INGREDIENTS

- Two 16-ounce bags dried navy or great Northern beans
- 1 cup light brown sugar, packed
- $\frac{1}{2}$ cup blackstrap molasses
- 2 tablespoons yellow mustard
- 2 tablespoons Dijon or whole-grained mustard

- 2 tablespoons tomato paste
- 2 tablespoons Worcestershire sauce
- 1 piece salt pork or fatback (about 2 inches square), cubed
- 6 strips bacon
- 1 onion, peeled and chopped

DIRECTIONS

1. At least 8 hours before cooking and baking the beans, pour them into a large bowl, add water to cover by about $\frac{1}{2}$ inch, and set aside to soak for at least 8 hours or overnight. The next day or when

you are ready to proceed with the dish, drain the beans and set aside momentarily.

2. Stir together the brown sugar, molasses, mustards, tomato paste and Worcester sauce in a small bowl.

3. Heat a large heavy-bottomed saucepan or Dutch oven over medium-high heat. Place the cubes of salt pork or fatback in the pan and sauté until browned and crisp. Remove and reserve the browned bits. Add the bacon to the pan and cook until golden brown and crisp. Remove the bacon to paper towels and drain all but about 3 tablespoons of the rendered fat from the pan, reserving the remaining fat.

4. Return the pan to medium-high heat, add the onion, and sauté until softened and golden brown. Stir in the reserved drained beans and brown sugar mixture and pour in water to just barely cover the beans. Reduce the heat to low, cover and simmer for one hour, stirring occasionally.

5. Meanwhile, preheat the oven to 250°F.

6. Pour the simmered beans into a large casserole dish, stir in the browned salt pork or fatback pieces, the remaining rendered fat (about $\frac{1}{4}$ cup), and crumble the browned bacon over top. Bake for about 40 minutes.

Just before serving the beans, remove any large pieces of salt pork or fatback.

PINEAPPLE SHERBET   MAKES 8 SERVINGS

Although most of my Richmond food memories center on my grandmother, pineapple sherbet puts me in mind of my grandfather. Throughout my childhood, he and I were pineapple sherbet buddies, and my fondness for the cold, creamy dessert has continued ever since.

Every day, my grandfather and I had the same routine. After dinner, I'd help my grandmother clean up in the kitchen for a few minutes and then make my escape to the porch. It was there that my grandfather—or Smokey, as I called him, because he was so big and dark—sat, relaxing in the rocking chair. I'd saunter over to the porch swing opposite him, all cool and nonchalant, and just wait. No more than 30 minutes would pass before he'd speak. "Lila," he'd say, breaking the silence, "I want you to go up to the High's and get me a quart of pineapple sherbet." Although he made the same declaration each night, Smokey spoke in an offhanded way that made this sound like a novel idea. I continued the ruse, answering, "Okay, Smokey," as I slowly brought the swing to a halt and stood up. He reached in his pocket for some money and, handing it to me said, "And get yourself a pint, too." The smile he offered shattered our little charade, and I darted off like a shot down the street to High's Ice Cream.

Traveling as quickly as possible with my arms full of sherbet, I returned only minutes later. I handed Smokey his quart, returned to the swing with my pint, and the two of us consumed the entirety of our respective containers in silent bliss. To this day, I can still imagine my grandmother in the kitchen, surrounded by piles of dirty dishes and smiling to herself. She knew Smokey and I were bonding on the porch over pineapple sherbet.

Smooth and creamy with chunks of juicy pineapple, the sherbet Smokey and I savored every day on his porch was perfection. In fact, on my return trips to Richmond as an adult, I always visited High's for my regular pint. As soon as the first spoonful of sherbet hit my lips, I was a little girl again sitting on Smokey's swing. The year I returned to Richmond to find that High's closed, I cried. Then I found another place to get sherbet.

Although the following recipe did not come from High's, it is pretty good, if I do say so myself. Because it is so simple, you really must use very ripe pineapple and either fresh or high-quality canned pineapple juice. Share this sherbet with someone you love, and make some memories of your own.

INGREDIENTS

- 2 cups Simple Syrup (see the recipe that follows)
- ½ cup chopped ripe pineapple
- 2 cups pineapple juice

DIRECTIONS

Combine all of the ingredients in a large bowl and freeze in an ice cream machine according to the manufacturer's directions. The sorbet should be soft and smooth, not hard and icy.

Serve with a spoon!

SIMPLE SYRUP
MAKES 2 CUPS

INGREDIENTS

- 2 cups sugar
- 1 cup water

DIRECTIONS

1. Combine the sugar and water in a medium saucepan, bring to a boil, and boil just until the sugar is melted.

2. Set aside to cool completely before using. Store the syrup in a sealed jar in the refrigerator or at room temperature.

Marjorie Jenkins, M.D.

Marjorie is the coauthor of *Eat Like a Woman*. She walks her talk—she exercises daily despite an extremely busy schedule, and she eats like a woman! You will love her flavorful Grilled Shrimp with Veggie Kabobs. Shrimp is low in saturated fat and a good source of niacin, iron, zinc and vitamin B_{12}. This meal is low calorie, high in protein, and easy to make—a perfect family meal.

As a team with her daughter Becca, she created super-delicious Low-Fat Banana Bread Muffins that are refreshingly simple to make and packed with I-want-to-eat-them-all temptation. Enjoy one and chew slowly so the creamy banana flavor satisfies your sweet tooth. Dr. Jenkins and Becca make a batch and freeze some for later—a good strategy for portion control!

GRILLED SHRIMP WITH VEGGIE KABOBS   MAKES 4 SERVINGS

This is a family favorite and a colorful, tasty meal during summer months when grilling is a mainstay.

INGREDIENTS

- 6 tablespoons olive oil, divided
- 4 teaspoons thyme, divided
- 3 teaspoons garlic powder, divided
- 2 teaspoons black truffle olive oil
- $\frac{1}{2}$ tsp salt (optional)
- 8 whole small sweet peppers (red, yellow and orange)
- 8 whole fresh cremini mushrooms
- Eight 2-inch chunks red onion
- 16 cherry tomatoes
- 1 pound small raw shrimp, not frozen or pre-cooked (40–60 count)

DIRECTIONS

1. **For the vegetable mix:** Mix 4 tablespoons of the olive oil, 3 teaspoons thyme, 2 teaspoons garlic powder, truffle oil and salt in a 9-by-13-inch pan or shallow bowl. Alternate peppers, mushrooms, onion and cherry tomatoes on a wooden or steel skewer and place in pan.

2. Using a basting brush, coat all sides of the vegetable kabobs with oil mixture. Set aside and brush again in 15 minutes.

3. **For the shrimp:** Mix 2 tablespoons of the olive oil, 1 teaspoon thyme and 1 teaspoon garlic powder, and mix with a fork or whisk. Pour over peeled shrimp and toss until shrimp are coated. Let shrimp sit for 15 minutes.

4. Turn grill on medium heat and place veggie kabobs on the grill. Rotate kabobs every 3 to 5 minutes and continue to cook until desired texture. Brush with remaining olive oil mixture from pan. We prefer 10 to 15 minutes, which keeps the veggies with just a hint of crispness.

5. In a grill pan throw shrimp on for 4 to 5 minutes only (do not overcook or they will be rubbery).

BECCA'S LOW-FAT BANANA BREAD MUFFINS   MAKES 24 MUFFINS

My daughter, Becca, is an aspiring chef. She also likes to eat healthy. We came up with this banana bread recipe, which is moist and flavorful. We like to make muffins because they bake quicker and we can freeze some for later.

INGREDIENTS

MUFFIN BASE:

- 3 to 4 ripe bananas
- $\frac{1}{4}$ cup low-fat sour cream
- 1 tablespoon canola oil
- 1 egg, beaten
- 1 cup sugar
- $1\frac{1}{2}$ cups flour
- $\frac{1}{4}$ teaspoon salt
- 1 teaspoon baking soda
- 1 teaspoon ground cinnamon
- $\frac{1}{2}$ teaspoon ground ginger
- $\frac{1}{4}$ teaspoon ground cloves
- $\frac{1}{4}$ cup toasted pecan pieces, at room temperature (optional)

TOPPING:

- $\frac{1}{2}$ cup packed brown sugar
- 2 teaspoons cinnamon

DIRECTIONS

1. Preheat the oven to 350°F. Mash the bananas in a bowl and add low-fat sour cream, oil and egg, and mix well until combined. Mix dry ingredients (sugar, flour, salt, baking soda, cinnamon, ginger and cloves) in a separate bowl until combined. Add dry ingredients to banana mixture. If using pecans, fold into batter.

2. Place muffin liners in tin and spray with nonstick cooking spray. Fill each to $\frac{2}{3}$ full of batter. Mix brown sugar with cinnamon. Sprinkle each muffin with the brown sugar cinnamon mixture.

3. Bake for 15 to 18 minutes in the center of the oven (cook times will vary based on altitude and oven). Bake until a toothpick inserted in center comes out clean.

Staness Jonekos

What foods you eat can make the difference between smooth life transitions or a bumpy road. Learning to eat like a woman is easy as you create new habits. The *Eat Like a Woman* Food Pyramid allows you the flexibility to eat delicious foods while improving your health and helping you find or maintain your healthy weight.

Balancing healthy foods with homemade treats is possible when you practice portion control. I have included a few of my favorite recipes to demonstrate how eating according to the food pyramid can still be incredibly satisfying and delicious.

Sprinkle in fun as you embrace eating like a woman! It is my hope that as you enjoy these recipes, it will fire up your imagination so you can create your own *Eat Like a Woman* recipes. Enjoy the dance with healthy food choices—bon appetit!

My Favorite Breakfasts

BAKED BREAKFAST FRITTATA   MAKES 6 TO 8 SERVINGS

This meal honors the *Eat Like a Woman* Food Pyramid—it is perfectly balanced, low in calories and the perfect way to start the day. The level of protein and fiber will keep you feeling full for hours.

INGREDIENTS

- 1 $\frac{1}{2}$ cups potatoes, cut in $\frac{1}{2}$ -inch cubes
- 1 tablespoon extra-virgin olive oil
- 1 $\frac{1}{2}$ cups cooked lean ham (8 ounces), chopped
- $\frac{3}{4}$ cup (3 ounces) low-fat shredded cheddar cheese, divided
- 8 eggs, slightly beaten (or two 8-ounce cartons of egg product)
- $\frac{1}{3}$ cup low-fat milk
- 2 chili peppers
- 2 teaspoons fresh oregano
- $\frac{1}{4}$ teaspoon salt
- One 4-ounce can diced green onions
- 2 teaspoons psyllium husks (you can buy this powdered fiber—it has no taste—at a health food store or grocery store such as Whole Foods)
- $\frac{1}{2}$ of a 7-ounce jar of roasted red sweet peppers, cut into thin strips
- 1 $\frac{1}{2}$ cups pre-made salsa
- $\frac{1}{4}$ cup fresh cilantro
- 3 sprigs parsley

DIRECTIONS

1. Preheat the oven to 350°F.

2. In a 10-inch oven-safe skillet, cook the potatoes in hot olive oil, uncovered, over medium heat for 5 minutes. Stir occasionally. Then cover and cook for another 5 minutes until tender. Remove from heat and mix in the ham and $\frac{1}{2}$ cup of cheddar cheese.

3. In a mixing bowl, stir together the eggs, milk, chili peppers, oregano, salt, onions and psyllium husks. Then pour into the skillet and mix together. Lay the pepper strips on top of the frittata.

4. Bake, uncovered, for 25 to 30 minutes.

5. Sprinkle the top with $\frac{1}{4}$ cup of cheddar cheese. In a separate pan, stir salsa and cilantro together and heat.

6. Cut the frittata into wedges, place the parsley as a decoration next to the wedge and serve with the salsa mixture. Serve on a smaller dish with a lovely wine glass filled with chilled water and a twist of lemon.

COFFEE MOCHA PROTEIN SHAKE MAKES ONE 8-OUNCE SERVING

INGREDIENTS

- 1 cup soy milk or skim milk
- 2 scoops whey chocolate protein powder
- 2 teaspoons instant coffee or a shot of espresso
- 1 teaspoon vanilla extract
- 1 cup ice cubes

DIRECTIONS

In a blender, combine all ingredients and blend until smooth. Enjoy!

Tip: You can pre-make this shake and refrigerate, and then pour it into an insulated thermos, so it will be ready to enjoy mid-afternoon.

My Favorite Lunches

CHICKEN CURRY SALAD MAKES 6 SERVINGS

Once you add the lettuce, pita or wrap, this meal honors the *Eat Like a Woman* Food Pyramid food ratios of 35 percent protein, 40 percent carbohydrates, and 25 percent fats.

By using curry, this scrumptious recipe contains enhanced health benefits. Curry is a blend of various spices, with the most common mixture being turmeric, ground cumin, cardamom and coriander. Curry boasts anti-inflammatory properties and can help promote neurological health.

With the addition of other healthy ingredients, such as onions, apples and chicken (an excellent lean meat choice), this salad is a healthy yet delicious way to jump-start your summer.

I like to serve this salad with sliced, chilled pears or apples on the side, and sparkling water with a sprig of mint...yummy!

INGREDIENTS

- ½ cup low-fat cottage cheese
- 1 teaspoon curry powder
- 1 dash pepper
- 2 large spring onions
- ¼ cup walnut halves, chopped
- 1 small apple, peeled and cubed
- 2 cups cooked chicken, breast meat only, chopped
- 1 head baby lettuce
- 6 mini whole-wheat pitas or wraps
- ¼ cup scallions, thinly sliced

DIRECTIONS

1. Puree the cottage cheese in a food processor. Add curry powder and pepper. Mix well. Puree to the desired consistency. I prefer a thicker puree, so I am careful not to over-process this mixture.

2. Add onions, walnut halves, apples and chicken to the curry mixture.

3. Serve on a bed of baby lettuce, or in ½ whole-wheat pita or wrap. Sprinkle thinly sliced scallions on top.

Serve chilled. Please note, it is best to make this recipe a few hours before serving. Sprinkle thinly sliced scallions on top.

TURKEY CHILI

MAKES 8 TO 10 SERVINGS

This is my all-time favorite chili recipe. The good news is that chili is not only comfort food, but it can be healthy, too!

Chili contains lots of protein. (This recipe is made with turkey, so it is a leaner alternative to ground beef.) And chili can help you lose weight. The capsaicin, a colorless compound found in the chilies used to season this dish, can increase your metabolic rate by increasing your body heat production. Chili is high in iron thanks to the turkey and beans, and it also has vitamin C thanks to the tomatoes, peppers and chilies. Plus, it's a great source of fiber that helps keep you full for a long time after eating. Enjoy the healthy benefits of chili!

INGREDIENTS

- 2 medium onions, chopped (1 cup)
- 1 tablespoon vegetable oil
- 2 tablespoons fresh garlic, chopped
- 1 medium green bell pepper, chopped (1 cup)
- 1 medium red bell pepper, chopped (1 cup)
- 2 pounds ground turkey
- 2 tablespoons ground cumin
- 1 tablespoon dried oregano leaves
- 1 tablespoon chili powder
- 1 can (4 ounces) chopped green chilies, drained
- 2 jalapeño chilies, seeded and chopped
- 1 can (28-ounce) whole Roma (plum) tomatoes
- 3 cups water for thick meaty chili, or 4 cups for "soupier" chili
- 2 cans (15 ounces) black beans, drained
- 1 can (15 to 16 ounces) kidney beans, drained
- Salt (to taste)
- Pepper (to taste)
- 1 sweet onion, sliced
- 1 tablespoon per serving low-fat sour cream

DIRECTIONS

1. Cook the onions in vegetable oil in a large saucepan over medium heat for about 10 minutes or until the onions are tender.

2. Add garlic and the green and red bell peppers; cook 2 to 3 minutes.

3. Add turkey and cook 3 to 4 minutes or until the turkey is no longer pink.

4. Add cumin, oregano, chili powder, green chilies, jalapeño chilies, tomatoes and water. Reduce heat to low.

5. Cover and simmer about 30 minutes.

6. Add beans; simmer 15 to 20 minutes longer. Season with salt and pepper. (I simmer for a total of 2 hours for a rich flavor.)

7. To serve, add sliced sweet onions to the top and a dab of low-fat sour cream.

If you want to make this recipe spicy, add one whole red habenero or one whole serrano chili (deveined, deseeded and chopped). Or if you like a Tex-Mex flavor, add an envelope of taco seasoning to the chili as it simmers.

My Favorite Dinners

ROMANTIC DINNER FOR TWO

This is a fun and romantic meal—ooh la la.

The menu:
Tempting beginning: Chilled grapes and fruit

Wine: Red (Zinfandel)

Main course: Chicken and Veggie Fondue with Dipping Sauces (low in fat and high in protein)

Sinful ending: Dark Chocolate Dipped Strawberries

CHICKEN AND VEGGIE FONDUE
WITH DIPPING SAUCES   MAKES 2 SERVINGS

INGREDIENTS

* 1 pound skinless and boneless chicken breasts
* 2 cups cauliflower
* 2 cups broccoli
* 4 ounces each of your favorite dipping sauces
* Vegetable oil

DIRECTIONS

1. For the chicken and veggies: Cut the chicken breasts and vegetables into bite-sized portions.

2. Place the chicken in a serving dish separate from the vegetables. Refrigerate until ready to serve.

3. Place your favorite dipping sauces in separate serving dishes.

Suggested dipping sauces: Peppercorn, honey mustard, peanut satay, sesame garlic, BBQ and/or teriyaki sauce. Purchase these sauces pre-made and keep your special evening simple.

4. **For the fondue:** Half fill the fondue pot with vegetable oil.

5. Pour the measured oil into a saucepan on the stovetop and heat the oil to 375°F. You will know the oil is ready when you drop a piece of bread in and it browns in 30 seconds.

6. Pour the oil back into the fondue pot and light the burner.

7. Place the chicken, vegetables and dipping sauces around the fondue pot.

8. Start cooking your dinner. Each piece of chicken should cook in the fondue pot 1 to 2 minutes.

DARK CHOCOLATE DIPPED STRAWBERRIES   MAKES 4 SERVINGS

After you have enjoyed cooking your fondue dinner, bring out the dark chocolate or chocolate-dipped strawberries for a sinful ending. Healthy dark chocolate has a cocoa content of 60 to 70 percent or higher. Eating 2 ounces (50 grams) a day of plain chocolate with a minimum content of 60 percent chocolate solids can be beneficial to health—providing protection against heart disease, high blood pressure, and many other health hazards, as well as providing vitamins and essential trace elements and nutrients such as iron, calcium and potassium. A 1 ½ -ounce square of chocolate may have as many cancer-fighting antioxidants as a 5-ounce glass of red wine. And chocolate stimulates the secretion of endorphins, producing a pleasurable sensation. So don't feel guilty—enjoy some dark chocolate!

INGREDIENTS

* 4 ounces semi-sweet dark chocolate

* 1 small carton medium-sized whole strawberries

DIRECTIONS

1. Microwave chocolate in a glass bowl, stopping after 30 seconds, then every 10 seconds until almost melted. Stir until smooth and glossy.

2. Wash strawberries and pat them dry (any moisture from the fruit will spoil the texture of the melted chocolate).

3. Dip each strawberry into the melted chocolate, covering the lower half of the strawberry.

4. Place on a baking sheet lined with wax paper.

5. Refrigerate for at least 1 hour.

TIPS FOR SELECTING YOUR WINE

The wine should not be sweeter than the chocolate you are serving.

When pairing wines with chocolate, the stronger the chocolate, the more full-bodied the wine should be. For example, a bittersweet chocolate tends to pair well with an intense Zinfandel.

Don't forget to play your favorite music, light plenty of candles and mist yourself with sensual perfume.

ROASTED TURKEY   MAKES 10 TO 12 SERVINGS

This recipe is perfect for entertaining or makes a great dinner for two with healthy leftovers.

INGREDIENTS

- 12–14 pound whole turkey, giblets removed
- 2 sprigs fresh thyme
- 2 sprigs oregano
- 2 sprigs sage
- 2 sprigs parsley
- 3 tablespoons olive oil

- 2 tablespoons dry white wine
- 2 tablespoons paprika
- Fresh ground pepper (to taste)
- 3 small oranges, unpeeled and cut into wedges
- 2 onions, cut into wedges
- 1 cup low-fat, low-sodium chicken broth

DIRECTIONS

1. Preheat the oven to 325°F.

2. Lift up the skin covering the turkey breast. Slip the thyme, oregano, sage and parsley underneath the skin.

3. Combine the oil, wine, paprika and pepper. Rub this mixture over the surface of the turkey.

4. Place the oranges and onions inside the turkey.

5. Place turkey, breast-side down, in a roasting pan. Pour chicken broth into the bottom of the pan. Cover loosely with aluminum foil.

6. Roast for 20 to 25 minutes per pound, basting periodically.

7. Halfway through cooking, place breast side up.

8. During last 45 minutes of roasting, remove cover.

9. Continue to roast until the leg moves easily and juices run clear.

10. Let stand for 20 minutes to let juices settle for easier carving.

My Favorite Sides and Snacks

LOW-FAT HUMMUS DIP
MAKES 10 TO 12 SERVINGS

INGREDIENTS

- 2 cans garbanzo beans, drained (and save the juice)
- 6 teaspoons lemon juice
- 4 tablespoons tahini
- 6 cloves garlic, peeled
- 1 teaspoon salt
- $\frac{1}{2}$ teaspoon pepper

DIRECTIONS

1. Combine all ingredients in a blender or food processor.

2. Process until smooth, and add the reserved garbanzo juice for a nice, creamy texture.

3. Serve with vegetables. Bell peppers, celery, cucumbers and carrots make a lovely and tasty presentation.

This recipe makes it possible to prepare two bowls of low-fat hummus, so you can have a presentation in the living room and one in the kitchen while guests keep you company during the turkey preparation.

ENDIVE, WATERCRESS AND PEAR SALAD
MAKES 10 TO 12 SERVINGS

INGREDIENTS

- 3 large bunches watercress, stems removed
- 3 heads Belgian endives, cored and separated into leaves
- 5 tablespoons extra-virgin olive oil
- Salt (to taste)
- Ground pepper (to taste)
- 3 tablespoons white balsamic vinegar (or pear vinegar)
- 3 ripe pears, halved and cored, then cut in half again lengthwise

DIRECTIONS

1. In a large bowl, toss watercress and Belgian endives.

2. Add extra-virgin olive oil and toss again.

3. Sprinkle with salt and freshly ground pepper and toss.

4. Pour in white balsamic vinegar, or pear vinegar, and then toss.

5. Garnish your salad with the pear wedges. Serve immediately.

My Favorite Dessert

BAKED APPLE PIE   MAKES 10 TO 12 SERVINGS

My husband shared this delicious recipe. It's an old family favorite!

INGREDIENTS

* 12 tart Jonathan apples
* 1 1/2 cups brown sugar
* 12 tablespoons light margarine (Smart Balance Light)
* 6 teaspoons ground cinnamon

DIRECTIONS

1. Preheat the oven to 350°F.

2. Core the apples but leave the bottom intact, so it looks like a "well" in the apple.

3. Prick the apple skins with a fork so the apple can "breathe" while baking.

4. Fill the hole with 2 tablespoons of brown sugar and 1 tablespoon of butter substitute.

5. Place the apples in a baking dish with a thin layer of water on the bottom, and sprinkle each apple with cinnamon.

6. Bake at 350°F for 20 minutes (10 minutes covered with foil and 10 minutes uncovered) until the apples are tender and begin to caramelize.

You can also add chopped walnuts or pecans to the "stuffing." And you may want to top this yummy recipe with a low-fat frozen vanilla yogurt.

APPENDIX A

HEALTHY PROTEINS, FATS, CARBOHYDRATES AND FIBER

Healthy Proteins

Lean poultry and fish are the best sources of protein with low calorie counts. Broil, bake, roast, steam or poach foods rather than fry them.

Fish and Seafood

- Cod
- Flounder
- Haddock
- Halibut
- Herring
- King crab
- Mackerel
- Mahi mahi
- Orange roughy
- Perch
- Pollock
- Salmon
- Sardines, in water
- Scallops
- Sea bass
- Shrimp
- Snapper
- Sole
- Tilapia
- Trout
- Tuna (canned in water)
- Wild catfish

Red Meat

- Flank steak
- Game meat: deer, elk
- Ground beef, extra lean
- London broil
- Pork chop
- Pork tenderloin
- Roast
- Top sirloin

White-Meat Poultry

Remove the skin before cooking.

- Chicken, light meat
- Game hen breasts
- Ground turkey, lean (98%)
- Turkey breast

Dairy and Eggs

- Camembert cheese
- Cheddar cheese, low fat
- Cottage cheese, low fat
- Egg Beaters
- Egg whites
- Eggs
- Greek yogurt, low fat
- Milk, skim or low fat
- Mozzarella, low fat
- Muenster cheese, low fat
- Parmesan cheese
- String cheese, low fat
- Swiss cheese, low fat
- Yogurt, low fat

Soy

Soy protein can help lower cholesterol and reduce the risk of heart disease.

- Soy burger and patty products
- Soy cheese
- Soy nuts
- Soybeans
- Tempeh
- Tofu

Beans

Beans and lentils are good sources of protein from high-fiber plant foods. They help you feel full for hours.

- Black beans
- Chickpeas
- Kidney beans
- Lentils
- Lima beans
- Navy beans

Nuts

Don't over-eat nuts because they're high in fat, too. Enjoy a small handful per day.

- Almonds
- Brazil nuts

- Cashews
- Peanuts

- Pistachios
- Walnuts

Protein Snacks for on the Go

- Cereal bar
- Cup of edamame
- Deli roll-up (turkey or chicken) with a slice of low-fat cheese (refer to "Dairy" list), add tomato and lettuce
- Energy bar (select one where carbohydrates and protein grams are about equal)
- Hard-boiled egg

- Meal-replacement drinks (watch out for sugar)—I enjoy Advantage's protein shakes and bars; they are high in protein and low in sugar. Watch those calories— if a bar is over 200 calories, cut it in half and enjoy the other half the next day.
- Pumpkin seeds (handful)
- String cheese
- Turkey jerky—be careful to avoid sodium- and sugar-filled brands

Healthy Fats

Monosaturated Fat

- Avocados
- Butters: almond, cashew, peanut, tahini/sesame paste, sunflower, hazelnut
- Canola oil
- Flaxseed oil

- Nuts: almonds, peanuts, pine nuts, walnuts, Brazil nuts, macadamia nuts, hazelnuts, pecans, cashews, pistachios
- Olive oil (extra virgin)
- Olives (black and green)
- Peanut oil

- Seeds: sesame, pumpkin, ground flaxseed, sunflower
- Sesame oil
- Soybean oil
- Sunflower oil
- Walnut oil

Polyunsaturated Fat

- Corn oil
- Cottonseed oil
- Flaxseed
- Flaxseed oil
- Fatty fish: salmon, tuna, mackerel, herring, trout, sardines
- Grape seed oil
- Pumpkin seeds
- Safflower oil
- Sesame seeds
- Soy milk
- Soybean oil
- Sunflower oil
- Sunflower seeds
- Tahini (sesame paste)
- Tofu
- Walnuts

TIPS

- Cook with olive oil. Use olive oil for stove-top cooking, rather than butter, stick margarine or lard. For baking, try canola or vegetable oil.
- You can add nuts to vegetable dishes or use them instead of breadcrumbs on chicken or fish.
- Dress your own salad. Commercial salad dressings are often high in saturated fat. Create your own healthy dressings with high-quality olive oil or sesame oil. Add condiments and spices, such as mustard, basil, ginger, garlic and cinnamon to increase flavor.

Healthy Carbohydrates Using the Glycemic Index (GI)

Low GI (55 or fewer)

CEREALS

- All Bran
- Oat Bran
- Rice Bran

BREADS

- 100% whole-grain wheat
- Nine-grain
- Oat bran
- Pumpernickel
- Spelt multigrain
- Three-grain sprouted grains

GRAINS

- Barley
- Buckwheat
- Bulgar

GLUTEN-FREE

+ Rice pasta, enriched

PASTA

+ Linguine
+ Vermicelli
+ Whole-wheat spaghetti

DAIRY

+ Milk (whole, low fat, or skim)
+ Soy milk
+ Yogurt

MILK ALTERNATIVES

+ Blue Diamond Unsweetened Chocolate Breeze (almond)
+ Vitasoy Light Original (soy milk)

FRUIT

+ Apple
+ Banana
+ Grapefruit
+ Grapes
+ Orange
+ Peach
+ Pear
+ Kiwi
+ Strawberries

VEGETABLES

+ Artichoke
+ Asparagus
+ Bean sprouts
+ Bok choy
+ Broccoli
+ Brussels sprouts
+ Cabbage
+ Carrots
+ Cauliflower
+ Celery
+ Cucumber
+ Eggplant
+ Green beans
+ Lettuce
+ Mushrooms
+ Onion
+ Peppers, red and green
+ Seaweed
+ Snow peas
+ Spinach
+ Squash
+ Sweet corn
+ Tomato (actually a fruit, cherry tomatoes are great in salads)
+ Water chestnuts, drained
+ Yam
+ Zucchini, raw

BEANS

- Black beans
- Kidney beans
- Lentils
- Navy beans
- Pinto beans
- Red beans
- Soybeans
- Split peas

NUTS AND SEEDS

- Almonds
- Cashews
- Flaxseeds
- Hazelnuts
- Macadamia nuts
- Peanuts
- Pecans
- Pine nuts
- Poppy seeds
- Pumpkin seeds, raw
- Sesame seeds
- Sunflower seeds
- Walnuts

Medium GI (56–70)

CEREALS

- Bran Chex
- Cream of Wheat
- Grape-Nuts
- Kashi 7 Whole Grain Puffs
- Life
- Muesli
- Oatmeal
- Puffed buckwheat
- Quaker Oats
- Quick Oats
- Raisin Bran
- Swiss muesli

BREADS

- Light rye bread
- Melba toast
- Organic stone-ground whole-wheat sourdough bread
- Pita bread
- Whole-wheat bread

GRAINS

- Couscous
- Rice, brown

PASTA

- Gnocchi, cooked
- Rice vermicelli noodles, dried, boiled
- Soba noodles/buckwheat noodles
- Udon noodles, plain, boiled

DAIRY

- Condensed milk, sweetened, full fat
- Ice cream

FRUIT

- Apricots
- Cantaloupe
- Cherries, dark
- Cranberries, dried, sweetened
- Figs, dried, tenderized
- Lychees, fresh
- Mango
- Papaya
- Pineapple
- Raisins

VEGETABLES

- Beets, canned
- Potatoes, boiled
- Potatoes, white, baked in skin
- Pumpkin, boiled
- Sweet potato

High GI (71 or more)

CEREAL

- Bran Flakes
- Cheerios
- Cocoa Krispies
- Corn flakes
- Crispix
- Grape-Nuts
- Rice Krispies
- Shredded Wheat

BREADS

- Bagel, white
- Baguette, traditional French bread
- Bread roll, white
- Gluten-free buckwheat bread
- Italian bread
- Kaiser roll, white
- Wonder white bread

GRAINS

- Jasmine rice, white, long-grain, cooked in rice cooker
- Millet
- Rice, instant

PASTA

* Rice pasta, brown, boiled
* Rice and corn pasta, gluten-free

FRUIT

* Lychees, canned, in syrup, drained
* Watermelon

VEGETABLES

* French fries
* Idahoan potatoes, instant, mashed
* Mashed potatoes, made with milk
* Parsnips
* Potato, baked, without skin
* Potato chips, deep fried
* Potatoes, new, unpeeled, boiled
* Potatoes, red, boiled, with skin
* Russet Burbank potatoes, baked, without fat
* Rutabaga

FACTORS THAT CAN AFFECT A FOOD'S GLYCEMIC INDEX

* FIBER CONTENT: The more fiber a food has, the less digestible carbohydrate, and so the less sugar it can deliver.
* PROCESSING: Grains that have been milled and refined have a higher glycemic index than whole grains.
* PHYSICAL FORM: Fincly ground grain is more rapidly digested, so it has a higher glycemic index than more coarsely ground grain.
* RIPENESS: Ripe fruits and vegetables tend to have more sugar than unripe ones, and so tend to have a higher glycemic index.

Healthy Fiber

Soluble

- Almonds
- Apples
- Barley
- Blueberries
- Brazil nuts
- Broccoli
- Flaxseed
- Lentils
- Lima beans
- Oat bran
- Oat cereal
- Oatmeal
- Oranges
- Peas
- Pears
- Psyllium seed husk
- Soybeans
- Strawberries
- Sweet potatoes (skins are also insoluble fiber)

Insoluble

- Brown rice
- Cauliflower
- Celery
- Green beans
- Nuts
- Root vegetable skins
- Wheat and corn bran
- Wheat bran
- Whole grains
- Whole wheat

APPENDIX B

SUPPLEMENTS, FOOD CHOICES AND RECOMMENDED DAILY ALLOWANCES PER LIFE STAGE

Your body was designed to absorb nutrients from food sources: consuming a healthy diet that includes natural food sources is the healthiest choice. Taking a daily multivitamin with minerals can be a good option if you are not consuming enough healthy foods.

Discuss all supplement choices with your health-care provider. Vitamins and minerals can affect your health if combined with certain drugs, and many medications deplete your body of essential nutrients. The following supplement chart is for women who are healthy.

Remember, dietary supplements cannot replace a healthy diet.

SUPPLEMENTS

Name	Body Benefits	Food Sources	Daily Dosage	General Information
Vitamin A	Treats skin disorders such as acne and good for eye health. There are some claims that there are antioxidant benefits. Vitamin A can also improve immune function.	Tuna fish, orange fruits (cantaloupe, mango, papaya, watermelon), dark-green and bright-colored veggies (broccoli, Brussels sprouts, carrots, kale, peas, pumpkin, spinach, sweet potato), pecans, pistachios, eggs, and dairy products (cheddar cheese, cow's milk, goat milk, goat cheese, sour cream)	700 micrograms (ages 14-70+) 750 micrograms (ages 14–18) during pregnancy 770 micrograms (ages 19–50) during pregnancy 1,200 micrograms (ages 14–18) during lactation 1,300 micrograms (ages 19–50) during lactation	Fat-soluble; stored in body. Do not take with blood thinners. Antacids and mineral oil may interfere with vitamin A absorption. Oral contraceptives are associated with increased blood levels of vitamin A.
Vitamin B$_1$ (Thiamine)	Good for the nervous system, muscle functioning, carbohydrate metabolism; aides with proper digestion; metabolizes carbohydrates.	Meat (pork loin, chicken breast, ground beef), legumes (pinto), whole grains, and seeds	1.0 milligrams (ages 14–18) 1.1 milligrams (ages 19+) 1.4 milligrams during pregnancy 1.4 milligrams during lactation	Water-soluble; excess is excreted in the urine. Large doses may cause drowsiness.

Name	Body Benefits	Food Sources	Daily Dosage	General Information
Vitamin B$_2$ Riboflavin	Necessary for normal cell function.	Organ meats, beef, salmon, tuna, chicken, turkey, eggs, milk, whole grains, buckwheat, oats, quinoa, green veggies (asparagus, broccoli, Brussels sprouts, spinach, broccoli, peas), beans (pinto, soy, navy, edamame), almonds and fruit (banana, grapes, lychee, mango, passionfruit)	1.0 milligram (ages 14–18) 1.1 milligrams (ages 19+) 1.4 milligrams during pregnancy 1.6 milligrams during lactation	Water-soluble; excess is excreted in the urine. Use caution if taking with herbs and other supplements with hormonal, diuretic or antidepressant activity. Oral contraceptives may reduce the conversion of B$_2$ to its active form.
Vitamin B$_3$ Niacin	Has been used to treat high cholesterol; may benefit age-related macular degeneration (AMD); promotes the conversion of food to energy.	Tuna (canned), chicken breast, ground beef (lean), enriched whole grains, barley, buckwheat, spelt, yeast, milk, eggs, veggies (artichoke, corn, mushrooms, peas, pumpkin, sweet potato), fruit (avocado, dates, guava, mango, nectarine, peach), edamame, split peas, soy beans and peanuts	14 milligrams (ages 14-70+) 18 milligrams during pregnancy 17 milligrams during lactation	Water-soluble; excess is excreted in the urine. B$_3$ can precipitate hot flashes in some women. Skin flushing to the face and neck may occur. Take with a meal to avoid gastrointestinal discomfort.

continued on page 258

Name	Body Benefits	Food Sources	Daily Dosage	General Information
Vitamin B$_5$ Panthothenic Acid	Essential to all life and to the metabolism of carbohydrates, proteins and fats, as well as the synthesis of hormones and cholesterol.	Brewer's yeast, organ meats, fish, shellfish, poultry, milk, eggs, whole grains, veggies (broccoli, Brussels sprouts, corn, mushrooms, sweet potato, squash, pumpkin), legumes (black-eyed peas, lima beans, soybeans, split peas), and fruit (avocado, dates, guava, raspberries, watermelon)	5 milligrams (ages 14-70+) 6 milligrams during pregnancy 7 milligrams during lactation	Water-soluble; excess is excreted in the urine. Drugs containing estrogen and progestin may increase your daily requirement.
Vitamin B$_6$ Pyridoxine	Required for the synthesis of the neurotransmitter, serotonin. Deficiency can affect nerves, skin, mucous membranes and the blood cell system.	Meat (ground beef), liver, tuna, salmon, chicken, turkey, fortified cereals, beans (kidney beans, lima beans, navy beans, soybeans, white beans), veggies (broccoli, raw carrots, Brussels sprouts, corn, green pepper, kale, okra, peas, sweet potato, potato with skin (baked), nuts (walnuts, chestnuts, hazelnuts), fruit (banana, grapes, guava, mango, pineapple, watermelon) and brown rice	1.2 milligrams (ages 14–18) 1.3 milligrams (ages 19–50) 1.5 milligrams (ages 51+) 1.9 milligrams during pregnancy 2.0 milligrams during lactation	Water-soluble; excess is excreted in the urine. Supplements with estrogen-like activity may interact with B$_6$.

Name	Body Benefits	Food Sources	Daily Dosage	General Information
Vitamin B$_9$ Folic Acid (also known as folate)	Often used to treat type 2 diabetes, high blood pressure, insomnia and restless leg syndrome.	Salmon, lamb, beef jerky, eggs, veggies (artichoke, asparagus, broccoli, cabbage, peas, spinach), brewer's yeast, cereals, fruit (blackberries, guava, orange, papaya, pineapple, raspberries, strawberries) and legumes (black-eyed peas, edamame, soybeans)	400 micrograms (ages 14-70+) 600 micrograms during pregnancy 500 micrograms during lactation	Water-soluble. Large doses of antacids can reduce folic acid absorption.
Vitamin B$_{12}$ Cobalamin	Helps maintain healthy nerve cells and red blood cells.	Fish (salmon, sardines, tuna, pollock, perch, herring, cod, caviar, catfish), oysters, crab, beef, pork, yogurt, ground chicken, eggs and dairy products (cheddar cheese, cottage cheese, cow's milk)	2.4 micrograms (ages 14-70+) 2.6 micrograms during pregnancy 2.8 micrograms during lactation	Water-soluble; excess is excreted in the urine. Excessive alcohol intake can decrease vitamin B$_{12}$ absorption. Supplemental vitamin C or iron may interfere with the bioavailability of vitamin B$_{12}$.

continued on page 260

Name	Body Benefits	Food Sources	Daily Dosage	General Information
Vitamin C	Necessary to form collagen in bones, cartilage, muscle and blood vessels. There is ongoing research on the use of vitamin C in the prevention or treatment of the common cold. There have been more than 30 clinical trials that showed no significant reduction in the risk of developing colds.	Fruits (grapefruit, strawberries, raspberries, guava, kiwi, mango, orange, papaya, pineapple), vegetables (broccoli, Brussels sprouts, green pepper, kale, tomato), fish (cod, perch), low-fat yogurt, soybeans and edamame	65 milligrams (ages 14–18) 75 milligrams (ages 19+) 85 milligrams during pregnancy 120 milligrams during lactation	Water-soluble; excess is excreted in the urine. High doses may cause diarrhea and nausea. Oral estrogens may decrease the effect of vitamin C in the body. Vitamin C increases iron absorption and may prolong clearance time for acetaminophen.
Vitamin D	Aides in the absorption of calcium, helping to form and maintain strong bones.	Egg yolks, liver, fish oils, fatty fish, fortified milk and fortified breakfast cereals In addition, 5 to 15 minutes of sunshine can boost vitamin D production.	600 IU (ages 1–70) 800 IU (ages 70+) 600 IU during pregnancy 600 IU during lactation	Fat-soluble. Intestinal absorption of vitamin D may be impaired with the use of mineral oil.

Name	Body Benefits	Food Sources	Daily Dosage	General Information
Vitamin E	Many people claim that vitamin E may prevent cardiovascular disease and cancer, but recent studies conclude that high doses of vitamin E (over 400 IU daily) may increase all-cause mortality and should be avoided.	Wheat germ oil, vegetables (broccoli, taro, butternut squash, potatoes parsnip), fruits (papaya, raspberries, peach, nectarine, mango, kiwi, guava, blueberries, blackberries), nuts and seeds (Brazil nuts, almonds, hazelnuts, pine nuts, sunflower seeds), fortified whole cereals, eggs, herring, sardines, turkey, edamame, pinto beans and butter	15 milligrams 15 milligrams during pregnancy 19 milligrams during lactation	Fat-soluble; can thin blood. Do not take with blood thinners without medical supervision. Caution that vitamin E doses over 400 IU/day are to be avoided in people taking warfarin and related anticoagulants because it interferes with platelet function.
Boron	May increase levels of certain estrogens.	Noncitrus fruits, leafy vegetables (broccoli), nuts (peanuts), dried fruit (raisins), avocado, legumes, wine, cider and beer	20 milligrams (ages 14-70+, pregnancy and lactation)	Overdose can cause nausea, vomiting, skin rash and diarrhea.

continued on page 262

Name	Body Benefits	Food Sources	Daily Dosage	General Information
Calcium/ Calcium Carbonate	Helps keep bones and teeth strong; maintains muscle and nerve functioning.	Milk, calcium-fortified orange juice, fortified cereals, yogurt, ricotta, nuts, tofu, kale, broccoli and spinach	1,300 milligrams (ages 9–18) 1,000 milligrams (ages 19–50) 1,300 milligrams (ages 14–18) during pregnancy 1,000 milligrams during pregnancy The same doses for lactation per age group 1,000 milligrams to 1,200 milligrams (all women ages 51+)	Must take with vitamin D for absorption.
Flaxseed	Can be used as a laxative. There are unproven claims that associate flaxseed with improved cardiovascular outcomes.	Purchase at health food store.	10–250 grams daily	Contains soluble fiber. Take with plenty of water. Do not take flaxseed at the same time as any conventional medication. It can lower the body's ability to absorb oral medications, and supplements. Take supplements 1–2 hours before taking flaxseed.

Name	Body Benefits	Food Sources	Daily Dosage	General Information
Magnesium	Helps maintain normal muscle and nerve function; keeps heart rhythm steady; supports a healthy immune system; keeps bones strong; helps to regulate blood sugar levels; promotes normal blood pressure; may manage disorders such as hypertension, cardiovascular disease and diabetes.	Fresh green veggies, spinach, beans, peas, nuts and seeds, fish, and whole unrefined grains	360 milligrams (ages 14–18) 310 milligrams (ages 19–30) 320 milligrams (ages 31+) 350 to 360 milligrams during pregnancy 310 to 320 milligrams during lactation	Helps with absorption of calcium. Taking some medicines, such as certain diuretics, antibiotics and medications taken to treat cancer, may result in magnesium deficiency.
Omega-3 and Omega-6 Fats	May assist in keeping triglyceride and cholesterol levels normal; can reduce the risk of nonfatal heart attacks and help reduce inflammation. Recent trials report a small reduction in blood pressure.	Fish oil, walnuts, vegetable oils (canola, soybean, flaxseed/linseed and olive oil), fish, herring, salmon, whitefish, tuna, bass, swordfish and sardines	1.1 grams* (ages 14-70+) 1.4 grams* pregnancy 1.3 grams* lactation 2–3 servings of fish weekly (salmon, trout, herring) *The Institute of Medicine daily Adequate Intake levels*	May add to the effects of drugs that may also affect blood pressure; can inhibit blood clotting. Consult with your doctor if taking Omega 3 & 6 and you have a chronic blood disorder.

continued on page 264

Name	Body Benefits	Food Sources	Daily Dosage	General Information
Phosphorus	Critical for energy storage, metabolism, the utilization of many B-complex vitamins, proper muscle and nerve function, and maintaining calcium balance.	Milk, cheese, dried beans, peas, colas, nuts, peanut butter	1,250 milligrams (ages 14–18) 700 milligrams (ages 19+) 700 milligrams during pregnancy and lactation	Potassium-sparring diuretics taken together with a phosphate may result in high blood levels of potassium.
Potassium	Necessary for the building of muscle, and for normal body growth; assists in carbohydrate metabolism; and controls body water balance.	Figs, apricots, banana, all meats, salmon, mushrooms, sunflower seeds, soy products, broccoli, peas, kidney beans, tomatoes, sweet potatoes, avocado, cantaloupe, kiwi, prunes, milk and yogurt	4,700 milligrams (ages 14-70+) 4,700 milligrams during pregnancy 5,100 milligrams during lactation	Diuretics, laxatives and steroids can cause loss of potassium.
Selenium	Demonstrates antioxidant properties; deficiency may affect thyroid function.	Liver, shellfish, salmon, tuna (canned), halibut, chicken breast (skinless), beef (lean), alfalfa, radish, onions, chives, brewer's yeast, wheat germ, butter, garlic, raisins, walnuts, cheddar cheese, eggs and sunflower seeds	55 micrograms (ages 14-70+) 60 micrograms during pregnancy 70 micrograms during lactation	Selenium levels may vary and may be related to estrogen status.

Name	Body Benefits	Food Sources	Daily Dosage	General Information
Zinc	May help keep the immune system functioning properly; necessary for the functioning of more than 300 different enzymes.	Legumes, meats, seafood, eggs, nuts, whole grains, oysters, sage and pumpkin seeds	30 milligrams daily for 14 days for immune function 9 milligrams (ages 14–18) 8 milligrams (ages 19–70) 11 milligrams during pregnancy 12 milligrams during lactation Upper tolerable limit 40 mg/day	May cause nausea, vomiting, or diarrhea. Zinc and penicillin bind, interfering with the absorption of one another. Zinc may reduce the absorption of tetracycline. Aspirin and oral contraceptives may decrease zinc status.

Supplement sources: National Academy of Sciences, National Institutes of Health, and the RDA (recommended dietary allowances, a collaborative effort between the USA and Canada).

If you have health concerns, such as kidney stones, high cholesterol, high blood pressure or heart disease, notify your doctor of any new supplements added to your daily plan. If you are taking high dosages of aspirin daily, consult your doctor before adjusting your supplements.

APPENDIX C

EAT LIKE A WOMAN MASTER FOOD CHART WITH FOOD BENEFITS

B = Brain health

DH = Digestive health

BH = Bone health

HH = Heart health

AI = Anti-inflammatory

AC = Anti-cancer

VG = Vegetarian (strict vegetarian: no red meat, poultry, seafood)

V = Vegan (no animal products, eggs, dairy, beeswax, honey, gelatin)

Food	B	DH	BH	HH	AI	AC	VG	V
Beverages								
Almond milk			X	X			X	X
Aloe vera juice		X			X		X	X
Coconut milk			X	X			X	X
Coffee (black)	X				X	X	X	X
Fresh-squeezed juices	X			X	X		X	X
Milk (nonfat, 2%, whole, lactose-reduced)			X					
Orange juice, fresh squeezed, calcium fortified	X	X	X	X			X	X
Red wine (1 serving)				X	X	X	X	X

Food	B	DH	BH	HH	AI	AC	VG	V
Rice milk				X			X	X
Soy milk, calcium fortified			X	X			X	X
Tea (green, black)	X			X	X	X	X	X
Water	X	X		X			X	X
Dairy								
Cheddar cheese			X					
Cheeses, low fat			X					
Cottage cheese, low fat	X		X					
Creamer, liquid (nondairy)							X	
Egg whites				X				
Eggs (omega-3s)	X		X	X		X (breast cancer)		
Ener-G egg replacement			X	X			X	X
Liquid eggs	X		X	X		X		
Margarine, fortified			X				X	
Milk (low fat and nonfat)	X		X	X				
Protein shake, fortified protein powder			X				X	X
Silk soy creamer			X	X			X	X
Soy cheese							X	
Soy milk			X	X			X	X
Swiss cheese			X					
Vegan cheese							X	X
Yogurt	X	X	X	X				

continued on page 268

Food	B	DH	BH	HH	AI	AC	VG	V
Fresh Fruit								
Apple	x	x	x	x	x	x	x	x
Apricot	x	x		x		x	x	x
Avocado		x		x	x	x	x	x
Banana	x	x	x	x			x	x
Blackberries		x		x	x	x	x	x
Blueberries	x	x		x	x	x	x	x
Cantaloupe		x		x	x		x	x
Cherries	x	x		x	x	x	x	x
Cranberries				x	x	x	x	x
Grapefruit		x	x		x		x	x
Grapes	x	x		x	x	x	x	x
Guava		x		x	x		x	x
Kiwi	x	x		x		x	x	x
Lemon					x		x	x
Lime					x		x	x
Mango		x		x	x	x	x	x
Mulberries					x			x
Orange		x	x	x	x	x	x	x
Papaya		x	x	x		x	x	x
Peach		x					x	x
Pear		x	x	x	x	x	x	x
Pineapple		x	x		x		x	x
Plum		x		x	x	x	x	x
Pomegranate		x	x	x		x	x	x
Prune			x			x	x	x
Raspberries		x		x	x	x	x	x
Strawberries		x	x		x	x	x	x
Watermelon		x		x		x	x	x

Food	B	DH	BH	HH	AI	AC	VG	V
Dried Fruit								
Apricots							X	X
Cherries				X			X	X
Dates		X		X			X	X
Figs		X	X	X		X	X	X
Prunes	X	X		X			X	X
Raisins		X	X				X	X
Breakfast Bars								
Advantage			X	X			X	
Cascadian Farm Granola				X			X	X
Luna Protein Bar			X				X	X
NuGo Bars Gluten free				X			X	X
ThinkThin Gluten free				X			X	X
Vegetables								
Artichoke		X	X	X		X	X	X
Asparagus	X	X	X	X	X		X	X
Beet				X		X	X	X
Bok choy		X	X	X	X	X	X	X
Broccoli		X	X	X	X	X	X	X
Brussels sprouts		X	X	X	X	X	X	X
Carrot		X		X	X		X	X
Cabbage	X	X	X	X		X	X	X
Cauliflower		X		X	X	X	X	X
Celery		X	X	X			X	X
Collard greens			X	X			X	X
Corn		X					X	X
Cucumber		X					X	X

continued on page 270

Food	B	DH	BH	HH	AI	AC	VG	V
Eggplant	X	X		X			X	X
Garlic		X		X	X	X	X	X
Green beans		X	X				X	X
Greens (kale, leek)			X	X	X		X	X
Lettuce		X		X			X	
Mushrooms		X	X	X		X	X	X
Olive		X			X		X	X
Onion		X	X	X			X	X
Peas			X	X			X	X
Peppers (green, red, yellow)			X	X			X	X
Spinach		X	X	X	X	X	X	X
Sprouts		X					X	X
Squash		X	X	X			X	X
Tomato		X	X	X	X		X	X
Zucchini					X		X	X
Grains								
100% whole-wheat bread (calcium fortified)		X	X	X			X	X
100% whole-wheat English muffin		X	X	X			X	X
100% whole-wheat pita		X	X	X			X	X
100% whole-wheat waffle		X	X	X			X	X
Bagel (white)		X		X			X	X
Barley		X		X	X		X	X
Bran and bran cereals		X		X			X	
Brown basmati rice		X		X			X	X
Brown rice		X		X		X	X	X
Brown rice bread		X		X			X	X

Food	B	DH	BH	HH	AI	AC	VG	V
Brown rice pasta		X		X			X	X
Buckwheat					X		X	X
Bulgar		X		X			X	X
Cereals: All Bran, Grape-Nuts, Shredded Wheat		X		X			X	X
Cereals: Kashi Heart Oatmeal, Cheerios, Life, Post Shredded Wheat		X	X	X			X	X
Flax crackers		X		X			X	X
Fortified cereals		X	X				X	X
Gluten-free waffles		X		X			X	X
Hot/cold cereals (calcium fortified)		X	X	X			X	
Millet	X	X					X	X
Oatmeal	X	X	X	X	X		X	X
Oats (steel cut)		X		X	X	X	X	X
Quinoa	X			X	X		X	X
Rye bread		X		X			X	X
Sprouted Ezekiel		X					X	X
Tortillas (corn flour)			X				X	X
Vegan breads		X		X			X	X
Wasa crackers		X					X	X
Wheat germ		X	X	X			X	X
Wheat grass		X					X	X
Wheat-free waffles		X		X			X	X
Whole-wheat pasta		X					X	X
Wild rice		X		X			X	X

continued on page 272

Food	B	DH	BH	HH	AI	AC	VG	V
Nuts and Seeds								
Almonds	X	X	X	X	X		X	X
Cashews		X		X	X	X	X	X
Flaxseeds		X		X	X		X	X
Hazelnuts				X	X		X	X
Macadamia nuts		X		X			X	X
Peanuts	X		X	X			X	X
Pecans				X		X	X	X
Pine nuts		X		X			X	X
Pistachios		X		X			X	X
Pumpkin seeds	X	X	X	X	X	X	X	X
Sesame seeds			X	X			X	X
Sunflower seeds	X				X		X	X
Walnuts	X	X		X	X	X	X	X
Tubers and Legumes								
Baked beans		X	X				X	X
Black beans		X		X		X	X	X
Garbanzo beans				X	X		X	X
Lentils		X		X	X		X	X
Pinto beans			X	X		X	X	X
Potatoes (white)							X	X
Red kidney beans			X	X		X	X	X
Russett potatoes						X	X	X
Split peas					X		X	X
Sweet potatoes		X	X	X	X		X	X
Soy								
Amy's Mexican Tofu Scramble			X	X	X	X	X	X
Breakfast patties/links			X	X	X	X	X	X

Food	B	DH	BH	HH	AI	AC	VG	V
Edamame			X	X	X	X	X	X
Miso			X	X	X	X	X	X
Soy patties			X	X	X	X	X	X
SoyBoy			X	X	X	X	X	X
Soyrizo			X	X	X	X	X	X
Tempeh			X	X	X	X	X	X
Tofu			X	X	X	X	X	X
Veggie burger patties			X	X	X	X	X	X
White beans			X	X			X	X
Yams		X		X			X	X
Fish and Seafood (wild is the best choice)								
Clams				X				
Cod				X	X			
Crab				X				
Haddock				X	X			
Halibut				X	X			
Lake trout				X	X			
Lobster								
Mahimahi				X				
Mussels				X				
Oysters					X			
Salmon	X		X	X	X			
Sardines (canned)			X	X	X	X		
Scallops				X				
Shrimp	X		X	X	X	X		
Sole				X				
Striped bass				X				

continued on page 274

Food	B	DH	BH	HH	AI	AC	VG	V
Tilapia				X	X			
Tuna			X	X	X			
Tuna (canned)	X		X	X	X			
Poultry (free-range is the best choice)								
Chicken (skinless)	X	X		X				
Cornish game hens	X			X				
Faux grilled chix				X			X	X
Lean ground turkey	X			X	X	X		
Lean turkey burgers	X			X	X	X		
Quail, pheasant	X			X	X			
Turkey (skinless)	X			X	X	X		
Turkey sausage	X			X	X			
Meat (grass-fed is the best choice)								
Beef (extra lean)				X				
Flank				X				
Lean ham				X				
Pork chop				X				
Pork tenderloin				X				
Roasts				X				
Top sirloin				X				
Wild game meats				X				
Meat Substitutes								
Meatless sausage links/meatballs		X		X			X	X
Veggie burgers		X		X			X	X
Oil and Seasonings								
Balsamic vinegar		X					X	X
Basil					X		X	X
Canola oil				X	X		X	X

Food	B	DH	BH	HH	AI	AC	VG	V
Cinnamon	X			X	X	X	X	X
Cloves					X		X	X
Coconut oil				X	X	X	X	X
Curry					X		X	X
Flaxseed oil				X	X		X	X
Ginger					X		X	X
Goat milk butter			X		X		X	
Hempseed oil				X			X	X
Mint		X					X	X
Mustard		X	X				X	X
Nutmeg	X			X			X	X
Olive oil (extra virgin)				X	X		X	X
Oregano					X		X	X
Organic butter					X		X	
Parsley					X	X	X	X
Peanut oil							X	X
Peppercorns		X		X		X	X	X
Red pepper flakes					X		X	X
Rosemary					X		X	X
Sesame oil				X			X	X
Thyme					X		X	X
Tumeric/cumin	X			X	X	X	X	X
Wine vinegar			X	X			X	X
Sweet Treats								
Dark chocolate	X			X	X			
Frozen low-fat yogurt		X		X				
Fruit sorbet		X		X			X	X
Graham crackers		X						

continued on page 276

Food	B	DH	BH	HH	AI	AC	VG	V
Rice Dream				x			x	x
Vegan chocolate							x	x
Vegan cookies							x	x
Extras								
Canned tomatoes		x	x	x	x		x	x
Frozen fruit		x		x	x	x	x	x
Frozen veggies		x		x	x	x	x	x
Hummus				x			x	x
Nut butters				x			x	x
Popcorn		x		x			x	x
Salsa				x			x	x
Soup (reduced sodium)				x			x	x
Vegan mayo							x	x

APPENDIX D

FOOD PLANS

How do you eat like a woman every day? I have created three sample food plans to get you started. You can enjoy the celebrity recipes in Chapter 14 for the first 2 weeks. If you love to eat, with no time to cook you will love the easy-to-follow food plan.

You can also combine recipes from different food plans and create your own program. If you have a busy day, select a daily menu from the "Love to eat, no time to cook." If you have a day with time and are in the mood to cook, choose from the celebrity recipes or the "Love to cook" food plan.

Just like selecting an outfit for the day, these food plans are like separates—pick and choose based on your mood and your schedule.

If you are like me, most of your days are busy and the "Love to eat, no time to cook" food plan will make food selections and preparation easy. Often I use these easy recipes and then select a fancy celebrity recipe for dinner.

Eating like a woman is all about celebrating health with delicious and nutritious food. Practice portion control on some of the easy-to-pig-out-on recipes like Hello Dolly Bars. Honor the *Eat Like a Woman* Food Pyramid, so you feel full for hours and fuel a healthy metabolism.

For additional recipes to create your own food plan, go to eatlikeawoman.com.

WEEK 1: *EAT LIKE A WOMAN* WITH CELEBRITY RECIPES

	Sunday	Monday	Tuesday	Wednesday	Thursday	Friday	Saturday
Breakfast	Breakfast burrito (scrambled eggs, cheddar cheese, black beans and salsa)	1-2 Chocolate-Chip Pancakes 2 fried eggs (p. 191)	Avocado Toast (p. 213) Hard-boiled egg	1 Becca's Low-Fat Banana Bread Muffin (p. 235) Protein shake	Low-fat cottage cheese with berries	Baked Breakfast Frittata (p. 236)	Oatmeal with protein powder and fruit
Snack *(optional if you eat breakfast more than 4 hours before lunch)*	100-calorie protein bar	Protein shake	Trail mix 1 low-fat string cheese	Celery with peanut butter	Pear with blue cheese and 1 Wasa crisp bread	$1\frac{1}{2}$ cups cantaloupe with 1 scoop low-fat cottage cheese	1 apple Greek yogurt
Lunch	Veggie burger (1 slice whole-wheat bread, lettuce and tomato)	Smoked Salmon and Wasabi Tea Sandwiches (p. 198)	Shake It Up Rice Salad with Grilled Lemon Chicken (p. 197)	Grilled Avocado Cobb Salad with Apricot Dressing (p. 201)	Tuna and Red Bean Salad (p. 220)	Tiny Tacos (p. 193)	Saturday Lunch Waldorf Chicken Salad (p. 213)
Snack	$\frac{1}{3}$ cup Grape-Nuts with 4 ounces low-fat Greek yogurt	Zesty Hot Nuts (small handful) (p. 214) 1 low-fat string cheese	Apple Crisp in a Mug (p. 224)	Low-Fat Hummus Dip with veggies	$\frac{1}{2}$ cup edamame	Coffee Mocha Protein Shake (p. 238)	Protein bar

	Sunday	Monday	Tuesday	Wednesday	Thursday	Friday	Saturday
Dinner	Simple Sunday Super Pot Roast (p. 215) Steamed veggies Free-Form Apple-Berry Tart (p. 216)	Broiled trout (rub with olive oil, salt & pepper, drizzle fresh lemon juice) Steamed veggies Brown rice Baked Apple Pie (p. 245)	Chinese Pepper Steak (p. 192) Grilled veggie of choice Fresh blueberries and strawberries with a sprinkle of sugar	Cat and Mo's Enchilada Pie (p. 202) No-Bake Dark Chocolate Ganache Tartlet (p. 203)	Honey-Glazed Pork Tenderloin (p. 194) Steamed green beans Brown rice Peaches in Red Wine (p. 223)	Two Hens Laughing (p. 222) Baked acorn squash Grasshopper cocktail (p. 199)	Steamed Blue Crabs (p. 229) Grilled Corn on the Cob (p. 230) Baked Beans (p. 231) Pineapple Sherbet (p. 232)
Snack	3.5 ounces red wine 1 low-fat string cheese	No snack if you eat the Baked Apple Pie (p. 245)	100-calorie protein bar	No snack if you eat the No-Bake Dark Chocolate Ganache Tartlet	No snack if you eat Peaches in Red Wine	Greek yogurt with berries	100-calorie protein bar

WEEK 2: *EAT LIKE A WOMAN* WITH CELEBRITY RECIPES

	Sunday	Monday	Tuesday	Wednesday	Thursday	Friday	Saturday
Breakfast	Baked Breakfast Frittata	Oat bran cereal, low-fat milk (or alternative) topped with fruit	Whole-wheat English muffin with soy sausage topped with melted, sliced low-fat cheese	2 to 3 ounces smoked salmon $\frac{1}{2}$ whole-wheat bagel	Poached egg, turkey sausage and whole-wheat toast	Gluten-free muesli with berries and Greek yogurt	1-2 Chocolate-Chip Pancakes (p. 191) Lean or meatless breakfast patty

continued on page 280

	Sunday	Monday	Tuesday	Wednesday	Thursday	Friday	Saturday
Snack *(optional if you eat breakfast more than 4 hours before lunch)*	½ cup steamed edamame	100-calorie protein bar	1 apple with 1 low-fat string cheese	Protein shake	Cataloupe with a scoop of cottage cheese	Turkey jerky	Cottage cheese with berries
Lunch	Tuna fish in whole-wheat pita with lettuce and tomato	Curried Orange Lentil Soup (p. 200)	Tuscan Kale and Heirloom Spinach Salad with grilled chicken (p. 228)	Chicken Curry Salad (p. 238)	Turkey Chili (p. 239)	Cool 'n' Crunchy Salmon Tacos (p. 225)	Tea Sandwiches with Goat Cheese and Cucumber (p. 221)
Snack	Leftover Tiny Tacos	1 low-fat string cheese with 6 almonds	Coffee Mocha Protein Shake (p. 238)	100-calorie protein bar	Celery with peanut butter	Hummus dip and veggies (p. 244)	Hard-boiled egg with melba toast
Dinner	Roasted turkey (p. 243) Baked squash Wild rice Baked Apple Pie (p. 245)	Mojo Criollo Slow-Braised Pork (p. 205) Brown Rice Steamed veggies Vegan-Chocolate-Mint Brownies (p. 206)	Striped Bass Tacos with Salsa Verde and Corn Peach Salsa (p. 209) Grilled green veggie Creamy Mango Cups (p. 211)	Three Amigos Guacamole with Grape Salsa (p. 218) Corn tortilla chips Margarita (I love Skinny Girl margaritas) Nancy's Mean Tortilla Soup (p. 196) Low-fat frozen yogurt	Endive, Watercress and Pear Salad Grilled Shrimp with Veggie Kabobs (p. 234) 1 Hello Dolly Bar (p. 227)	Romantic Dinner for Two (p. 241), including Dark Chocolate Dipped Strawberries (p. 242)	Filet mignon topped with peppercorns and blue cheese Smashed Yukon Gold Potatoes (p. 207) Phyllo Cups with Greek Yogurt, Fresh Peaches and Honey (p. 208)

	Sunday	Monday	Tuesday	Wednesday	Thursday	Friday	Saturday
Snack	Cottage cheese and fruit	No snack if you eat the Vegan Chocolate-Mint Brownies	No snack if you eat the Creamy Mango Cups	1 low-fat string cheese with a handful of pumpkin seeds	No snack if you eat the Hello Dolly Bar	100-calorie protein bar	Greek yogurt with berries

THE "LOVE TO EAT, NO TIME TO COOK" FOOD PLAN

	Sunday	Monday	Tuesday	Wednesday	Thursday	Friday	Saturday
Breakfast	Baked Breakfast Fritatta (p. 236)	½ cup fruit with ½ cup low-fat cottage cheese coffee	½ cup oatmeal with 1 tablespoon protein powder ½ cup fruit ½ cup soy milk in coffee	Protein shake	1 egg, hardboiled with 3 ounces lean ham coffee	½ cup fruit with ½ cup cottage cheese coffee	4 ounces low-fat yogurt coffee
Mid-morning snack	½ cup fruit with ½ cup cottage cheese	100-calorie protein bar	½ protein shake	½ cup fruit with ½ cup cottage cheese	100-calorie protein bar	½ protein shake	100-calorie protein bar

continued on page 282

	Sunday	Monday	Tuesday	Wednesday	Thursday	Friday	Saturday
Lunch	Turkey salad: 6 ounces turkey with lettuce, veggies and low-fat dressing	1 cup veggies with 6 ounces grilled chicken	4 ounces of tuna on $\frac{1}{2}$ pita pocket with light mayo $\frac{1}{2}$ cup fruit	1 cup lean turkey chili (p. 239) with 1 medium apple	4 ounces crabmeat in $\frac{1}{2}$ pita pocket with 1 teaspoon light mayo	Chicken salad: 6 ounces grilled chicken with lettuce and veggies	6 ounces lean ground beef with 1 cup veggies
Afternoon Snack	2 hard-boiled eggs stuffed with hummus, sprinkle paprika for spice	String cheese with medium apple	1 ounce cashews	Coffee Mocha shake (p. 238)	1 ounce macadamia nuts	4 ounces tuna, light mayo, 2 melba toasts	Low-fat string cheese with $\frac{1}{2}$ cup fruit
Dinner	Stir-fry chicken and veggies with small salad	6 ounces pork chop with 1 cup veggies	6 ounces grilled salmon with 1 cup veggies	6 ounces grilled chicken with 1 cup veggies	6 ounces white fish with 1 cup veggies	6 ounces beef tenderloin with salad with low-fat dressing 6 ounces red wine	Chicken and Veggie Fondue (see Romantic Dinner for Two recipe (p. 241)) 6 ounces white wine
Evening Snack	100-calorie protein bar	Low-fat yogurt	4 ounces red wine and low-fat string cheese	1-2 ounces turkey lunch meat with small apple	Protein shake	Fruit with low-fat string cheese	Fruit with low-fat yogurt

TIPS FOR ALL *EAT LIKE A WOMAN* FOOD PLANS:

* Six ounces of red wine can be enjoyed at dinner—substitute for the yam, brown rice or bread serving *or* decrease portion size of carb.

* One cup of black coffee or green tea can be consumed at breakfast. Use only low-fat or nonfat dairy milk, or soy or almond milk, and no sugar.

EAT LIKE A WOMAN RULES:

* Eat within 1 hour of waking (if you wake up early, have a mid-morning snack).

* Have lunch within 4 hours of breakfast.

* Have your mid-afternoon snack 3 to 4 hours after lunch.

* Have dinner no later than 3 hours after snack.

* The nighttime snack should be consumed 1 hour before bedtime.

* If you go to work or out of the house during the day, take a snack pack with your food prepared.

* Never skip breakfast!

* Eat slowly and drink water with your meals. Lemon in your water or tea helps speed up your metabolism.

* Watch your portion sizes. Remember, if the food group is bigger than your fist, you are over consuming.

* Carry snacks with you at all times.

For a shopping list, visit eatlikeawoman.com.

APPENDIX E

EAT LIKE A WOMAN-APPROVED HEALTHY SNACKS AND HEALTHY FAST FOOD CHOICES

More than 25 percent of calorie intake each day for Americans is composed of snacks, according to the Institute of Food Technologies, a nonprofit scientific society. Since 1977, snacking has become a fourth meal, averaging 580 calories a day, with beverages accounting for 50 percent.

Eat Like a Woman defines a healthy snack as less than 150 calories. Sugar is not listed as the first ingredient, and fat is less than half the total calories. You want protein and fiber to keep you feeling full.

Here are some tips on selecting healthy snacks:

+ Aim for fruits, vegetables and whole-grain snacks.
+ Naturally sweetened is better than foods and drinks that contain added sugar.
+ Choose low-fat or fat-free options.
+ Fresh fruit is a healthier choice than a fruit-flavored drink. Foods and drinks that list sugar or corn syrup as one of the first ingredients are not healthy snack choices.

Healthy Snacks

Fruit
* 1 medium apple (dried or cut into wedges, great with cinnamon)
* 1 small banana
* ¼ cup raisins
* 1 cup strawberries

Vegetables
* A dozen baby carrots
* Snap peas (the pods are edible)
* Celery sticks (add some peanut butter)
* 1 cup raw cauliflower
* 1 cup grape tomatoes
* ¼ cup hummus with veggies

Dairy
* 1 oz low-fat cheddar cheese
* ½ cup fat-free or low-fat milk
* ½ cup low-fat cottage cheese
* 6-8 ounces low-fat or fat-free plain yogurt
* 1 stick low-fat string cheese

Bread, cereal, rice and pasta
* 3 cups air-popped popcorn (sprinkle Parmesan cheese or chili powder instead of salt)
* 2 brown rice or multigrain rice cakes
* 2 Graham crackers
* ⅓ cup Grape-Nuts with 4 ounces of nonfat plain vanilla yogurt
* Oatmeal, stir in nuts

Protein
* Chicken slices
* Edamame, soy milk, tofu or toasted soybeans—vegan friendly
* Hard-boiled egg
* Jerky (meatless options available)
* Turkey slices

Other
* Homemade trail mix (handful)
* Nuts—lima beans, cashews, almonds, walnuts (small handful or 10 nuts)
* Protein bars (100-200 calories)
* Protein shake (100-200 calories)
* ½ cup pumpkin seeds in shell

Healthy Fast Food Choices

Here are some tips on selecting healthy fast food options:

* Drink water instead of a soda or shake.
* Avoid deep-fried, batter-dipped, breaded, creamy and crispy foods.
* Order without mayo or request low-fat mayo.
* Use low-fat dressings for salads. Ask for olive oil and vinegar or order dressing on the side and spoon on a small amount.
* Avoid sour cream, cheese and spreads.
* Avoid super-sized portions or value-sized choices.
* Avoid bacon—instead, add extra pickles, onions, lettuce, tomatoes and/or mustard.
* Veggie burgers are a great meatless option and a lower calorie option—but watch the sauces and spreads.
* Order skinless chicken without breading; grilled chicken is a good choice.
* Order black beans instead of refried beans.
* Chinese food: order egg drop, wonton or hot-and-sour soup, and get steamed brown rice instead of white. Use low-sodium soy sauce.

Arby's
* Grilled Chicken Caesar
* Martha's Vineyard Salad
* Roasted Chicken Salad

Blimpie
* Turkey & Provolone Sandwich

Burger King
* Chucky Chicken Salad
* BK Broiler Chicken Sandwich
* BK Veggie Burger (hold mayo—vegan option)

Carl's Jr.
* Charbroiled BBQ Chicken Sandwich
* Charbroiled Chicken Salad-To-Go

Chick-fil-A

- Chargrilled Chicken Garden Salad
- Chargrilled Chicken Sandwich

Chipotle

- Burrito Bowls (skip the tortilla)

Jack in the Box

- Asian Chicken Salad with Grilled Chicken Strips
- Chicken Fajita Pita

Kenny Roger's Roasters

- Chicken Caesar Salad
- Roasted Chicken Salad
- Half Chicken without skin
- Sliced Turkey Breast

KFC

- Original Recipe Sandwich without sauce
- Tender Roast Sandwich
- Roasted Caesar Salad
- Tender Roast Sandwich without sauce

Long John Silver's

- Grilled Chicken Salad

McDonald's

My first paycheck came from McDonald's, and I am happy to report that they have some good, healthy options.

- Apple Slices
- Grilled Chicken Snack Wrap
- Egg McMuffin
- Premium Asian Salad with grilled chicken
- Fruit and Maple Oatmeal
- Fruit and Yogurt Parfait
- Southwest Salad with grilled chicken (use ½ dressing or bring your own)
- Grilled Chicken Salad

Panera Bread

- Black Bean Soup and Mediterranean Veggie Sandwich
- Half Turkey Artichoke on Focaccia Bread with a bowl of Black Bean Soup (or garden salad, low-fat dressing)

Subway

Order 6" subs with whole-wheat bread. Eat only half of the bread (open faced) and request low-fat mayo; Swiss or mozzarella cheese are better choices. You can also use low-fat dressing or mustard instead of mayo.

- Honey Mustard Turkey with Cucumber
- Roast Beef
- Roasted Chicken Breast
- Roasted Chicken Salad
- Turkey Breast
- Veggie Delight (hold the mayo & cheese—vegan option)

Taco Bell

- Bean Burrito (replace cheese with fresh salsa—vegan option)
- Fresco Crunchy Taco
- Fresco Style Ranchero Chicken Soft Taco
- Grilled Chicken Burrito

Wendy's

- Grilled Chicken Sandwich
- Mandarin Chicken Salad
- Small Chili
- Ultimate Chicken Grill

Source: USDA National Nutrient Database for Standard Reference, US Department of Agriculture, USDA Food Composition Data, Release 14.

APPENDIX F

EXERCISE AND CALORIES BURNED PER HOUR

Exercise	Calories Burned per Hour			
	130 lbs	155 lbs	180 lbs	205 lbs
Aerobics, general	384	457	531	605
Aerobics, high impact	413	493	572	651
Aerobics, low impact	295	352	409	465
Aerobics, step aerobics	502	598	695	791
Archery	207	246	286	326
Backpacking, hiking with pack	413	493	572	651
Badminton	266	317	368	419
Bagging grass, leaves	236	281	327	372
Bakery, light effort	148	176	204	233
Ballet, twist, jazz, tap	266	317	368	419
Ballroom dancing, fast	325	387	449	512
Ballroom dancing, slow	177	211	245	279
Basketball, playing, non-competitive	354	422	490	558
Basketball, shooting baskets	266	317	368	419
Bathing dog	207	246	286	326
Bird watching	148	176	204	233
Bowling	177	211	245	279

continued on page 290

Exercise	Calories Burned per Hour			
	130 lbs	155 lbs	180 lbs	205 lbs
Boxing, in ring	708	844	981	1,117
Boxing, punching bag	354	422	490	558
Boxing, sparring	531	633	735	838
Calisthenics, light: pushups, situps	207	246	286	326
Calisthenics, fast: pushups, situps	472	563	654	745
Canoeing, camping trip	236	281	327	372
Canoeing, rowing, light	177	211	245	279
Canoeing, rowing, moderate	413	493	572	651
Canoeing, rowing, vigorous	708	844	981	1,117
Carrying 16 to 24 lbs, up stairs	354	422	490	558
Carrying 25 to 49 lbs, up stairs	472	563	654	745
Carrying heavy loads	472	563	654	745
Carrying infant, level ground	207	246	286	326
Carrying infant, up stairs	295	352	409	465
Carrying moderate loads, up stairs	472	563	654	745
Carrying small children	177	211	245	279
Children's games (e.g., hopscotch)	295	352	409	465
Circuit training, minimal rest	472	563	654	745
Cleaning gutters	295	352	409	465
Climbing hills, carrying up to 9 lbs	413	493	572	651
Climbing hills, carrying 10 to 20 lbs	443	528	613	698
Climbing hills, carrying 21 to 42 lbs	472	563	654	745
Climbing hills, carrying over 42 lbs	531	633	735	838
Crew, sculling, rowing, competition	708	844	981	1,117
Cricket (batting, bowling)	295	352	409	465
Croquet	148	176	204	233
Cross-country skiing, slow	413	493	572	651
Cross-country skiing, moderate	472	563	654	745

Exercise	Calories Burned per Hour			
	130 lbs	155 lbs	180 lbs	205 lbs
Cross-country skiing, racing	826	985	1,144	1,303
Cycling, <10 mph, leisure bicycling	236	281	327	372
Cycling, >20 mph, racing	944	1,126	1,308	1,489
Cycling, 10-11.9 mph, light	354	422	490	558
Cycling, 12-13.9 mph, moderate	472	563	654	745
Cycling, 14-15.9 mph, vigorous	590	704	817	931
Cycling, 16-19 mph, very fast, racing	708	844	981	1,117
Cycling, mountain bike	502	598	695	791
Darts (wall or lawn)	148	176	204	233
Diving, springboard or platform	177	211	245	279
Downhill skiing, moderate	354	422	490	558
Farming, feeding horses or cattle	266	317	368	419
Farming, feeding small animals	236	281	327	372
Fencing	354	422	490	558
Fishing from boat, sitting	148	176	204	233
Fishing from riverbank, standing	207	246	286	326
Fishing from riverbank, walking	236	281	327	372
Fishing in stream, in waders	354	422	490	558
Fishing, general	177	211	245	279
Fishing, ice fishing	118	141	163	186
Football or baseball, playing catch	148	176	204	233
Football, touch, flag, general	472	563	654	745
Frisbee playing, general	177	211	245	279
Frisbee, ultimate frisbee	472	563	654	745
General cleaning	207	246	286	326
Golf, driving range	177	211	245	279
Golf, general	266	317	368	419
Golf, miniature golf	177	211	245	279

continued on page 292

Exercise	Calories Burned per Hour			
	130 lbs	155 lbs	180 lbs	205 lbs
Golf, using power cart	207	246	286	326
Golf, walking and pulling clubs	254	303	351	400
Golf, walking and carrying clubs	266	317	368	419
Gymnastics	236	281	327	372
Handball	708	844	981	1,117
Handball, team	472	563	654	745
Health club exercise	325	387	449	512
Hiking, cross country	354	422	490	558
Hockey, field hockey	472	563	654	745
Hockey, ice hockey	472	563	654	745
Horse grooming	354	422	490	558
Horse racing, galloping	472	563	654	745
Horse racing, trotting	384	457	531	605
Horse racing, walking	153	183	212	242
Horseback riding	236	281	327	372
Horseback riding, grooming horse	207	246	286	326
Horseback riding, saddling horse	207	246	286	326
Horseback riding, trotting	384	457	531	605
Horseback riding, walking	148	176	204	233
Horseshoe pitching	177	211	245	279
Housework, light	148	176	204	233
Housework, moderate	207	246	286	326
Housework, vigorous	236	281	327	372
Ice skating, <9 mph	325	387	449	512
Ice skating, average speed	413	493	572	651
Ice skating, rapidly	531	633	735	838
Instructing aerobic class	354	422	490	558
Jai alai	708	844	981	1,117

Exercise	Calories Burned per Hour			
	130 lbs	155 lbs	180 lbs	205 lbs
Jazzercise	354	422	490	558
Judo, karate, jujitsu, martial arts	590	704	817	931
Juggling	236	281	327	372
Jumping rope, fast	708	844	981	1,117
Jumping rope, moderate	590	704	817	931
Jumping rope, slow	472	563	654	745
Kayaking	295	352	409	465
Kick boxing	590	704	817	931
Kickball	413	493	572	651
Loading, unloading car	177	211	245	279
Mowing lawn, riding mower	148	176	204	233
Music, playing a cello	118	141	163	186
Music, playing drums	236	281	327	372
Music, playing guitar	177	211	245	279
Music, playing piano	148	176	204	233
Music, playing trombone	207	246	286	326
Music, playing trumpet	148	176	204	233
Music, playing violin	148	176	204	233
Paddle boat	236	281	327	372
Paddleball, competitive	590	704	817	931
Paddleball, playing	354	422	490	558
Painting	266	317	368	419
Polo	472	563	654	745
Pushing a wheelchair	236	281	327	372
Pushing stroller, walking with children	148	176	204	233
Race walking	384	457	531	605
Racquetball, competitive	590	704	817	931
Racquetball, playing	413	493	572	651

continued on page 294

Exercise	Calories Burned per Hour			
	130 lbs	155 lbs	180 lbs	205 lbs
Rock climbing, ascending rock	649	774	899	1,024
Rock climbing, mountain climbing	472	563	654	745
Rock climbing, rappelling	472	563	654	745
Roller blading, in-line skating	708	844	981	1,117
Roller skating	413	493	572	651
Rowing machine, light	207	246	286	326
Rowing machine, moderate	413	493	572	651
Rowing machine, very vigorous	708	844	981	1,117
Rowing machine, vigorous	502	598	695	791
Running, 5 mph (12-minute mile)	472	563	654	745
Running, 5.2 mph (11.5-minute mile)	531	633	735	838
Running, 6 mph (10-minute mile)	590	704	817	931
Running, 6.7 mph (9-minute mile)	649	774	899	1,024
Running, 7 mph (8.5-minute mile)	679	809	940	1,070
Running, 7.5 mph (8-minute mile)	738	880	1,022	1,163
Running, 8 mph (7.5-minute mile)	797	950	1,103	1,256
Running, 8.6 mph (7-minute mile)	826	985	1,144	1,303
Running, 9 mph (6.5-minute mile)	885	1,056	1,226	1,396
Running, 10 mph (6-minute mile)	944	1,126	1,308	1,489
Running, 10.9 mph (5.5-minute mile)	1,062	1,267	1,471	1,675
Running, cross country	531	633	735	838
Running, general	472	563	654	745
Running, on a track, team practice	590	704	817	931
Running, up stairs	885	1,056	1,226	1,396
Sailing, competition	295	352	409	465
Sailing, yachting, ocean sailing	177	211	245	279
Shuffleboard, lawn bowling	177	211	245	279
Sitting, playing with animals, light	148	176	204	233

Exercise	Calories Burned per Hour			
	130 lbs	155 lbs	180 lbs	205 lbs
Sitting, light office work	89	106	123	140
Ski mobiling	413	493	572	651
Skiing, water skiing	354	422	490	558
Skin diving, fast	944	1,126	1,308	1,489
Skin diving, moderate	738	880	1,022	1,163
Skin diving, scuba diving	413	493	572	651
Skydiving	177	211	245	279
Snorkeling	295	352	409	465
Snow shoeing	472	563	654	745
Snow skiing, downhill skiing, light	295	352	409	465
Snowmobiling	207	246	286	326
Soccer, playing	413	493	572	651
Softball or baseball	295	352	409	465
Softball, pitching	354	422	490	558
Squash	708	844	981	1117
Stair machine	531	633	735	838
Standing, playing with children, light	165	197	229	261
Stationary cycling, light	325	387	449	512
Stationary cycling, moderate	413	493	572	651
Stationary cycling, very light	177	211	245	279
Stationary cycling, very vigorous	738	880	1,022	1,163
Stationary cycling, vigorous	620	739	858	977
Steel mill, working in general	472	563	654	745
Stretching, hatha yoga	236	281	327	372
Stretching, mild	148	176	204	233
Surfing, body surfing or board surfing	177	211	245	279
Swimming backstroke	413	493	572	651
Swimming breaststroke	590	704	817	931

continued on page 296

Exercise	Calories Burned per Hour			
	130 lbs	155 lbs	180 lbs	205 lbs
Swimming butterfly	649	774	899	1,024
Swimming laps, freestyle, fast	590	704	817	931
Swimming laps, freestyle, slow	413	493	572	651
Swimming leisurely, not laps	354	422	490	558
Swimming sidestroke	472	563	654	745
Swimming synchronized	472	563	654	745
Swimming, treading water, fast	590	704	817	931
Swimming, treading water, moderate	236	281	327	372
Table tennis, ping pong	236	281	327	372
Tae kwan do, martial arts	590	704	817	931
Tai chi	236	281	327	372
Taking out trash	177	211	245	279
Tennis, playing	413	493	572	651
Tennis, doubles	354	422	490	558
Tennis, singles	472	563	654	745
Track and field (high jump, pole vault)	354	422	490	558
Track and field (hurdles)	590	704	817	931
Track and field (shot, discus)	236	281	327	372
Trampoline	207	246	286	326
Typing, computer data entry	89	106	123	140
Using crutches	295	352	409	465
Volleyball, playing	177	211	245	279
Volleyball, beach	472	563	654	745
Volleyball, competitive	472	563	654	745
Walk/run, playing, moderate	236	281	327	372
Walk/run, playing, vigorous	295	352	409	465
Walking 2.0 mph, slow	148	176	204	233
Walking 2.5 mph	177	211	245	279

Exercise	Calories Burned per Hour			
	130 lbs	155 lbs	180 lbs	205 lbs
Walking 3.0 mph, moderate	195	232	270	307
Walking 3.5 mph, brisk pace	224	267	311	354
Walking 3.5 mph, uphill	354	422	490	558
Walking 4.0 mph, very brisk	295	352	409	465
Walking 4.5 mph	372	443	515	586
Walking 5.0 mph	472	563	654	745
Walking downstairs	177	211	245	279
Walking the dog	177	211	245	279
Walking, under 2.0 mph, very slow	118	141	163	186
Water aerobics	236	281	327	372
Water aerobics, water calisthenics	236	281	327	372
Water jogging	472	563	654	745
Water volleyball	177	211	245	279
Watering lawn or garden	89	106	123	140
Weeding, cultivating garden	266	317	368	419
Weight lifting, body building, vigorous	354	422	490	558
Weight lifting, light workout	177	211	245	279
Whitewater rafting, kayaking, canoeing	295	352	409	465
Windsurfing, sailing	177	211	245	279

TYPES OF ACTIVITIES AND INTENSITY (REPETITIVE)
(1 minute of vigorous activity equals 2 minutes of moderate activity)

CATEGORY	INTENSITY	TYPE OF EXERCISE
Aerobic	Moderate	Walking fast (3 mph or faster) Doubles tennis Water aerobics Biking level terrain (slower than 10 mph) Ballroom dancing General gardening
	Vigorous	Jogging Swimming laps Biking on hills (faster than 10 mph) Singles tennis Basketball Hiking uphill Heavy gardening Jumping rope Zumba
Muscle-strengthening		Lifting weights Yoga Using resistance bands Dumbbells Use your body weight (plank pose)

If you are doing a moderate-intensity activity, you can talk, but not sing, during the activity. If you are doing a vigorous-intensity activity, you will not be able to say more than a few words without pausing for a breath.

HELPFUL WEBSITES

FOR *EAT LIKE A WOMAN*-APPROVED RECIPES, HEALTH CALCULATORS, PHONE APPS, AND SUPPORT

- Eat Like a Woman: www.EatLikeAWoman.com

WOMEN'S HEALTH

- Center for the Study of Sex Differences in Health, Aging, and Disease: www.csd.georgetown.edu
- European Society of Gender Health and Medicine: www.gendermedicine.org
- Gender and Health Collaborative Curriculum Project—Canada: www.genderandhealth.ca
- Gendered Innovations: www.genderedinnovations.standford.edu
- Institute for Gender Health Canada: www.cihr-irsc.gc.ca/e/8673.html
- International Menopause Society: www.imsociety.org
- The North American Menopause Society: www.menopause.org
- Know the Difference: www.KnowTheDifferences.com
- Laura W. Bush Institute for Women's Health at Texas Tech University Health Sciences Center: www.laurabushinstitute.org
- Office on Women's Health: www.WomensHealth.gov
- Organization for the Study of Sex Differences: www.ossdweb.org
- Sex and Gender Women's Health Collaborative: www.sgwhc.org
- Society for Women's Health Research: www.swhr.org
- The International Society for Gender Medicine: www.isogem.com
- Women's Health Research Institute at Northwestern University: www.womenshealth.northwestern.edu

NUTRITION INFORMATION

- Academy of Nutrition and Dietetics: ww.eatright.org
- Dietary Guidelines for Americans: www.health.gov/dietaryguidelines/dga2005/healthieryou/contents.htm
- Food and Nutrition Service, USDA: www.fns.usda.gov/
- Fooducate nutrition app makes shopping for healthy foods easier: www.fooducate.com
- Gateway to Government Food Safety Information: www.FoodSafety.gov
- Herbalgram.org: www.herbalgram.org/
- How to read food labels: www.fda.gov/Food/IngredientsPackagingLabeling/LabelingNutrition/ucm079449.htm
- International Food Information Council Foundation: www.foodinsight.org
- Linus Pauling Institute (information on vitamins, minerals & phytonutrients): www.lpi.oregonstate.edu
- National Institutes of Health, Office of Dietary Supplements: www.ods.od.nih.gov/
- Nutrition.gov: www.Nutrition.gov
- NuVal System, provides comprehensive nutritional information: www.nuval.com/
- USDA Food and Nutrition Information Center (FNDIC): fnic.nal.usda.gov
- Vegetarian Resource Group: www.vrg.org/

SUPPORT BY CONDITION

- Academy for Eating Disorders: www.aedweb.org
- The American Cancer Society: www.cancer.org
- American Diabetes Association: www.diabetes.org/
- American Gastroenterological Association: www.gastro.org
- American Heart Association: www.americanheart.org
- American Heart Association Food Certification Program: www.checkmark.heart.org
- American Psychological Association: www.apa.org
- Celiac Disease Foundation: www.celiac.org
- Eating Disorders Anonymous: www.eatingdisordersanonymous.org
- The Food Allergy and Anaphylaxis Network: www.foodallergy.org
- National Association of Anorexia Nervosa and Associated Disorders: www.anad.org

- National Association to Advance Fat Acceptance: www.naafa.org
- National Digestive Diseases Information Clearinghouse, NIDDK, NIH, HHS: www.digestive.niddk.nih.gov
- National Stroke Association: www.stroke.org
- National Heart, Lung, and Blood Institute: www.nhlbi.nih.gov/
- National Institute of Mental Health, NIH, HHS: www.nimh.nih.gov
- Overeaters Anonymous: www.oa.org
- T.H.E. (Treatment, Healing, Education) Center for Disordered Eating: www.thecenternc.org
- Weight-Control Information Network: www.win.niddk.gov

HEALTH AND SAFETY RESOURCES

- American College of Sports Medicine: www.acsm.org/
- American Council on Science and Health (ACSH): www.acsh.org
- Centers for Disease Control and Prevention: www.cdc.gov/foodsafety
- Connects people with leading medical experts: MedHelp.org
- Consumer Reports: www.consumerreports.org
- Database on health topics: MedlinePlus.gov
- Division of Nutrition, Physical Activity and Obesity, CDC: www.cdc.gov/nccdphp/dnpa/
- National Center for Complementary and Alternative Medicine (CAM): www.nccam.nih.gov/
- U.S. Environmental Protection Agency Office of Water: www.epa.gov/OW
- U.S. Food and Drug Administration: www.fda.gov
- USDA Nutrient Data Laboratory: www.Ndb.nal.usda.gov/ndb/foods/list

POPULAR CONSUMER HEALTH WEBSITES

* Health and wellness social media platform that connects people with top-ranking experts created by Dr. Oz and Jeff Arnold: www.sharecare.com
* Nation's leading independent health information resource: www.healthywomen.org/
* Nonprofit organization that helps people 50 and older: AARP.org
* Relevant content to promote a healthy lifestyle: Healthline.com
* Social health company for women: www.empowher.com

PARTICIPATE IN A CLINICAL TRIAL

* www.nih.gov/health/clinicaltrials/findingatrial.htm

BOOK REFERENCES

* www.eatlikeawoman.com/footer/book-references/

AUTHORS' NOTE

Eat Like a Woman reveals remarkable sex differences, but it is only the beginning, a small step in the march for women's health. We must support science so women have a future that includes health management based on our biological sex differences.

It took millions of women (and men) campaigning for breast cancer research—because our voices were heard there are advances in early detection, and better treatment and management options today.

Join us and support science that acknowledges sex differences—it benefits both sexes.

The Society for Women's Health Research (SWHR) is a nonprofit organization and the thought leader in research on biological differences in disease.

Donate today and help improve health for all women through increased research, advocacy and public education programs that expand our understanding of women's unique needs in all areas of health.

Thanks to SWHR's advocacy and public policy efforts, women's health issues are now a *national* priority.

Visit www.SWHR.org, click "donate" on the top bar, and make a difference today.

ACKNOWLEDGMENTS

Born during the women's rights movement, I was part of the first generation to benefit from the efforts of many courageous women who demanded more from life. I had freedoms my mother never knew.

I had the right to choose marriage, children, education and career. I assumed all women's rights had been "handled" until I hit menopause and realized women's health was still in its infancy.

After writing my first book, *The Menopause Makeover,* with women's health expert Wendy Klein, M.D., my world changed. Wendy Klein gave me a golden ticket to a new universe, and I will forever feel blessed that I call Wendy my friend, and I am so thankful women like her are making sure women's health receives equal attention.

Committed to my new passion, Wendy connected me to another leader in women's health and expert in sex-based science—Marjorie Jenkins, M.D. Coauthor Dr. Jenkins shared her vast knowledge and expertise in a way that was fun. We are all fortunate that she is part of a coalition demanding that sex-based science is practiced, and I am lucky that one of the smartest women out there partnered with me to make sure the information in this book is accurate and that I had access to the latest women's health science. I will be forever grateful.

Without the skilled efforts of my literary agent, Rick Broadhead, *Eat Like a Woman* would not have been born. Rick is the classiest agent out there. His grace in managing projects has made each book a true joy.

You hear stories about people wanting to write a book, but they never do—it is only a dream. Deb Brody, editorial director at Harlequin Nonfiction, made my dream come true. She has a gift for finding passion and chiseling something beautiful out of it. But most of all, I will be forever grateful for her compassion and support during my father's final months.

Jacqueline, talent booker extraordinaire, was responsible for securing our favorite celebrity recipes included in this book. Thank you for your incredible enthusiasm and fearlessness—it's great to work with a pro.

A big thank-you to Sally Stewart, who inspired this book with her genius idea to call my food program *Eat Like a Woman*.

To each of the super star celebrities and chefs, thank you for supporting *Eat Like a Woman* with your recipes. I am proud this book shares the message that being healthy can taste *great*!

A dear friend who has shared her God-given artistic talent and friendship on all of my projects, Bethany Berndt-Shackelford, I thank you for bringing color and design into my life.

Landon Lung, technical wizard and master of all things in the cyber world, thank you for keeping me online in style!

I want to thank my brother, Stan Jonekos II, for always cheering me on. And my mother, Joyce Jonekos, who taught me to go out and get what I want, because she did not have the same opportunities until recently—thank you.

To all my girlfriends who dragged me out for dinner so I would not forget there is life on the other side of the computer monitor. Thank you to my long-time buddy Sara Martin for always believing in my projects and offering to help when I was slammed with deadlines. Terri Seifried, thank you for being my go-to expert with the celebrity recipes and sharing great conversations about food science.

I know my husband, Michael Becker, is reading this and saying, "Hey, what about me, the guy who supported and loved you during this entire process that included looking at you at the computer 10 straight months, 10 hours a day?" Well, baby, I wanted to save the best for last. Being married to you has made it possible to live my dreams, but most important, being loved by you makes me the luckiest girl in the world. Your passion to create and make the world a better place inspires me every day. I love you forever.

INDEX

ABOUT THE AUTHORS

Staness Jonekos is an award-winning television writer, producer and director, as well as an author and writer on women's health issues.

She was one of the original executive producers who launched the television network Oxygen Media, cofounded by Oprah Winfrey. Following her commitment to health, Staness co-executive produced the premiere season of VH1's *Celebrity Fit Club,* and post-produced Lifetime's *Speaking of Women's Health.* She is the president and founder of Krystal Productions, a film and video production company based in Los Angeles.

In addition to her extensive work experience behind the camera, Staness is a tireless advocate for women's health, wellness and empowerment. Her first book, *The Menopause Makeover,* was a pioneering work in the field of menopause, a highly visual and inspiring survival guide that challenged the conventional, old-style approach to managing menopause.

She has appeared on the *Today* show, contributes to the *Huffington Post,* and has been featured in a variety of publications ranging from the *Houston Chronicle* to More.com.

After college, Staness appeared on *The Love Boat, Falcon's Crest,* and *The Young and the Restless,* as well as cohosting *Shop Television Network.*

Staness holds a bachelor's degree in theater from UCLA and is an active member of the Producers Guild of America, the Academy of Television Arts & Sciences, the International Documentary Association, the North American Menopause Society, the Academy of Women's Health, and the International Menopause Society.

Planning an escape strategy from Los Angeles, Staness looks forward to writing her next book in the country, enjoying new adventures with her husband, Michael; their German shepherd, Salem; and their newly adopted Brittany spaniel, Rye.

Marjorie Jenkins, M.D., F.A.C.P., is a Professor of Medicine and Associate Dean for Women in Health and Science at the Texas Tech University Health Science Center (TTUHSC) where she holds the J Avery "Janie" Rush Endowed Chair for Excellence in Women's Health. At TTUHSC she works with a group of talented faculty and students in developing the first U.S. medical school, pharmacy school and nursing school curricula in sex and gender medicine. She is engaged nationally and serves as an executive council member of the Sex and Gender Women's Health Collaborative, a member of the Women's Health Task Force of the National Board of Medical Examiners, a founding board member for the Academy of Women's Health, and an expert panel member for the Health Resources and Services Administration *Women's Health Curricula: Report on Interprofessional Collaboration Across the Health Professions.*

Possessing a unique combination of skills, with her passion as the driving force, Dr. Jenkins wrote a proposal to then First Lady Laura W. Bush to create the Laura W. Bush Institute for Women's Health (LWBIWH) at Texas Tech University Health Sciences Center. The LWBIWH is dedicated to research and education focused on sex and gender differences. Stemming from Dr. Jenkins' leadership, the Laura W. Bush Institute at TTUHSC was established and has expanded to five cities in West Texas. TTUHSC is a leading voice in moving forward the national and international conversation about the clear need for researchers, physicians, nurses, pharmacists and students who are aware of the health differences between the female and male genders.

By invitation, Dr. Jenkins has delivered in excess of 100 presentations to professional and public audiences and coauthored numerous works in both the scientific and public arenas. She has been honored with many awards, such as Soroptimist's "Woman of the Year," the Business and Professional Women's "Texas Women to Watch," and the Hispanic Chamber of Commerce's "Taking Care of Our Own." She has been recognized with the TTUHSC President's Community Engagement Award, the TTUHSC School of Medicine's Most Published Faculty and is a 2013 Texas SuperDoc. In addition, Dr. Jenkins continues to find the time to educate men and women through her radio show via KGNC News Talk 710 and on her blog, www.knowthedifferences.com.

Dr. Jenkins and her husband, Steve, are parents to three wonderful children, Katharine, Matthew and Rebecca. Living in an environment so in tune to gender differences, Dr. Jenkins's children often have spirited conversations about sex and gender differences over dinner. Spare time allows Dr. Jenkins to enjoy biking, and she and Steve enjoy cooking exciting and diverse foods for family and friends.

When asked for a summation as to why it is imperative for sex and gender differences to be integrated throughout the world, Dr. Jenkins flashes a telling smile that lets whomever asked know that a statement of conviction is to follow. Her reply: "You have to know the difference to make a difference!"